T0326317

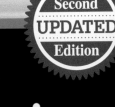

Second **UPDATED** **Edition**

Curbside Consultation in Oculoplastics

49 Clinical Questions

Curbside Consultation in Ophthalmology

SERIES

SERIES EDITOR, DAVID F. CHANG, MD

Curbside Consultation in Oculoplastics

49 Clinical Questions

EDITORS

Robert C. Kersten, MD, FACS
Professor of Clinical Ophthalmology
University of California San Francisco Medical School
San Francisco, California

Timothy J. McCulley, MD
Vice Chair for Clinical Strategic Planning
Director, Fellowship in Oculoplastics
Director, Division of Neuro-ophthalmology
Wilmer Eye Institute
Johns Hopkins School of Medicine
Baltimore, Maryland

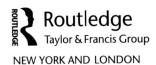

Routledge
Taylor & Francis Group

NEW YORK AND LONDON

First published 2016 by SLACK Incorporated

Published 2024 by CRC Press
2385 NW Executive Center Drive, Suite 320, Boca Raton FL 33431

and by CRC Press
4 Park Square, Milton Park, Abingdon, Oxon, OX14 4RN

CRC Press is an imprint of Taylor & Francis Group, LLC

Library of Congress Cataloging-in-Publication Data

Curbside consultation in oculoplastics : 49 clinical questions / [edited by] Robert C. Kersten, Timothy J. McCulley. -- Second edition.
    p. ; cm. -- (Curbside consultation)
  Includes bibliographical references and index.
  ISBN 9781617119170 (alk. paper)
  I. Kersten, Robert C., editor. II. McCulley, Timothy J., editor. III. Series: Curbside consultation in ophthalmology series.
  [DNLM: 1. Ophthalmologic Surgical Procedures. 2. Eyelids--surgery. 3. Reconstructive Surgical Procedures. WW 168]
  RE87
  617.7'1--dc23
                        2015018377

ISBN: 9781617119170 (pbk)
ISBN: 9781003523604 (ebk)

DOI: 10.1201/9781003523604

Dedication

I have been very fortunate to have had many mentors, partners, colleagues, and fellows who have helped teach me and have kept me thinking throughout my years in ophthalmology. They are too many to name, but I would like to dedicate this book to the spirit of friendship and fellowship we have all enjoyed. A special thanks, though, should go to my mentor, Richard Anderson, and to my friends and colleagues, Jeff Nerad, Ed Holland, and Jerry Popham, with whom I have especially enjoyed working over the years.

Robert C. Kersten, MD, FACS

This book is dedicated to my wife, Lynda, and children, Dean, Amelia, and Dylan, who generously share my time and attention with various academic pursuits, including book editing.

Timothy J. McCulley, MD

Contents

About the Editors

Robert C. Kersten, MD, FACS is Professor of Ophthalmology at University of California San Francisco School of Medicine. He has trained more than 30 postgraduate fellows in oculofacial plastic surgery and authored more than 100 peer-reviewed publications and 30 textbook chapters. He is a member of the Orbit Society and has served on the editorial boards of numerous scientific journals dealing with ophthalmic plastic surgery. He lectures widely on an international basis and has received the Senior Honor Award from the American Academy of Ophthalmology, where he served as editor of the Basic and Clinical Science Course series on Orbit, Eyelids, and Lacrimal System.

Timothy J. McCulley, MD is the Vice Chair of Clinical Strategic Planning, Primary Preceptor for an American Society of Oculoplastic and Reconstructive Surgery (ASOPRS) Accredited Fellowship, and Director of the Division of Neuro-ophthalmology at the Wilmer Eye Institute, Johns Hopkins School of Medicine. In 1995, he obtained his medical degree at Washington University School of Medicine in St. Louis. After a combined medical and surgical internship at the University of Hawaii, he completed residency in ophthalmology at Stanford University in 1999. Following 1 year of fellowship training in neuro-ophthalmology at the Bascom Palmer Eye Institute, he completed 2 years of fellowship training in ophthalmic plastic and reconstructive surgery at the Cincinnati Eye Institute in 2003. Dr. McCulley was on faculty at Stanford University, where he served as director of both neuro-ophthalmology and oculoplastic surgery. In 2006, he relocated to the University of California San Francisco, where he served as Director of Oculoplastic Surgery and as the primary preceptor for an (ASOPRS) fellowship. Dr. McCulley joined the Wilmer Eye Institute in 2011 and spent 2 years as director of ophthalmic plastic and reconstructive surgery at King Khaled Eye Specialist Hospital (KKESH), Wilmer's affiliate hospital in Saudi Arabia. He returned to Maryland in 2013. This is the second edition of the second book edited by Dr. McCulley. He has also contributed to more than 20 book chapters and authored more than 75 peer-reviewed manuscripts.

Contributing Authors

Gary L. Aguilar, MD (Question 16)
San Francisco, California

Bishr Al Dabagh, MD (Question 22)
Michigan Dermatology
Flint, Michigan

Elizabeth A. Atchison, MD (Question 26)
Resident in Ophthalmology
Department of Ophthalmology
Mayo Clinic
Rochester, Minnesota

Michèle Beaconsfield, DO, FRCS, FRCOphth,
    FEBO (Question 21)
Consultant Ophthalmic & Oculoplastic Surgeon
Moorfields Eye Hospital
London, United Kingdom

Linda C. Chang, MD (Question 22)
Assistant Professor
University of Washington
Seattle, Washington

William Chen, MD (Question 4)
Clinical Professor of Ophthalmology
Harbor-UCLA Medical Center
Torrance, California
UCLA School of Medicine
Los Angeles, California

Richard Collin, MA, FRCS, FRCOphth, DO
    (Question 21)
Honorary Professor of Ophthalmology
    UCL & Consultant Ophthalmic Surgeon
    Moorfields Eye Hospital
London, England

Murray Cotter, MD, PhD (Question 22)
Dermatology Associates of North Michigan
Petoskey, Michigan

Roger A. Dailey, MD, FACS (Question 2)
Lester T. Jones Endowed Chair
Chief, Casey Aesthetic Facial Surgery Center
    & Thyroid Eye Disease Clinic
Oculofacial Plastic Surgery Division &
    Department of Dermatology
Past President, American Society of Ophthalmic
    Plastic & Reconstructive Surgery
Oregon Health & Sciences University
Portland, Oregon

Steven C. Dresner, MD (Question 12)
Clinical Professor
USC Keck School of Medicine and USC Eye
    Institute
Los Angeles, California

Vikram D. Durairaj, MD (Question 30)
Oculoplastic and Orbital Surgery
Director, ASOPRS Fellowship
Texas Oculoplastic Consultants
Austin, Texas

Bita Esmaeli, MD, FACS (Question 41)
Professor of Ophthalmology
Director, Ophthalmic Plastic & Reconstructive
    Surgery Fellowship Program
Department of Plastic Surgery
University of Texas MD Anderson Cancer Center
Houston, Texas

Daniel G. Ezra, MA, MBBS, MMedEd, MD,
    FRCS, FRCOphth (Question 39)
Consultant Ophthalmic Surgeon
Adnexal Service, Moorfields Eye Hospital
Honorary Lecturer in Ophthalmology
Moorfields and UCL Institute of Ophthalmology
NIHR Biomedical Research Centre
London, England

James A. Garrity, MD (Question 26)
Professor of Ophthalmology
Department of Ophthalmology
Mayo Clinic
Rochester, Minnesota

Robert Alan Goldberg, MD (Question 18)
Chief, Orbital and Ophthalmic Plastic Surgery
UCLA Stein Eye Institute
Professor of Ophthalmology
David Geffen School of Medicine at UCLA
Los Angeles, California

Karl C. Golnik, MD, MEd (Question 25)
Professor
Departments of Ophthalmology, Neurology, and Neurosurgery
University of Cincinnati & the Cincinnati Eye Institute
Cincinnati, Ohio

Heidi M. Hermes, MD, FAAD (Question 23)
Harrison HealthPartners Dermatology
Sequim, Washington

Marc J. Hirschbein, MD, FACS (Question 34)
Director
Aesthetic Eyelid and Facial Surgery
Associate Chairman
Krieger Eye Institute
Baltimore, Maryland

Catherine J. Hwang, MD (Question 15)
Assistant Clinical Professor
Associate Physician Diplomate
Division of Orbital & Ophthalmic Plastic Surgery
Jules Stein Eye Institute/UCLA
Los Angeles, California

Thomas N. Hwang, MD, PhD (Question 45)
Staff Physician
The Permanent Medical Group
Redwood City, California

Thomas E. Johnson, MD (Question 42)
Professor of Clinical Ophthalmology
Bascom Palmer Eye Institute
University of Miami Miller School of Medicine
Miami, Florida

David R. Jordan, MD, FACS, FRCSC (Question 47)
Professor of Ophthalmology
University of Ottawa Eye Institute and the Ottawa Hospital
Ottawa, Ontario, Canada

James A. Katowitz, MD (Question 13)
Professor Emeritus and Director of Oculoplastic and Orbital Surgery
The Children's Hospital of Philadelphia and The Edwin and Fannie Gray Hall Center for Human Appearance
Perelman School of Medicine
The University of Pennsylvania

William R. Katowitz, MD (Question 13)
Assistant Professor of Clinical Ophthalmology
The Children's Hospital of Philadelphia and The Edwin and Fannie Gray Hall Center for Human Appearance
Perelman School of Medicine
The University of Pennsylvania
Philadelphia, Pennsylvania

Michael Kazim, MD (Question 37)
Clinical Professor of Ophthalmology and Surgery
Columbia University Medical Center
New York, New York

Don O. Kikkawa, MD (Question 43)
Professor of Clinical Ophthalmology
Chief, Division of Ophthalmic Plastic and Reconstructive Surgery
Vice Chair, Department of Ophthalmology
University of California, San Diego
La Jolla, California

Jane S. Kim, MD (Question 43)
Division of Ophthalmic Plastic and Reconstructive Surgery
Department of Ophthalmology
University of California, San Diego
La Jolla, California

Jonathan W. Kim, MD (Question 28)
Director, Ocular Oncology
Associate Professor of Ophthalmology
USC Keck School of Medicine
Los Angeles, California

Audrey C. Ko, MD (Question 6)
Bascom Palmer Eye Institute
University of Miami Department of
  Ophthalmology
Miami, Florida

Marcus J. Ko, MD (Question 6)
Nevada Centre Eye Plastic Surgery
Reno, Nevada

Bobby S. Korn, MD, PhD (Question 24)
Associate Professor of Ophthalmology and
  Plastic Surgery
University of California, San Diego School of
  Medicine
La Jolla, California

Andrea Lora Kossler, MD (Question 31)
Assistant Professor of Ophthalmology
Director, Ophthalmic Plastic, Reconstructive
  Surgery & Orbital Oncology
Byers Eye Institute at Stanford University
Stanford School of Medicine
Stanford, California

Andrew G. Lee, MD (Question 48)
Chair, Department of Ophthalmology
Houston Methodist Hospital
Adjunct Professor of Ophthalmology
Baylor College of Medicine
University of Texas MD Anderson Cancer Center
Houston, Texas
Clinical Professor of Ophthalmology
The University of Texas Medical Branch
Galveston, Texas
Professor of Ophthalmology, Neurology, and
  Neurosurgery
Weill Cornell Medical College
New York, New York
Adjunct Professor of Ophthalmology
The University of Iowa Hospitals and Clinics
Iowa City, Iowa

Bradford W. Lee, MD, MSc (Question 24)
Assistant Professor of Ophthalmology
Bascom Palmer Eye Institute
University of Miami School of Medicine
Palm Beach Gardens, Florida

N. Grace Lee, MD (Question 17)
Instructor in Ophthalmology
Harvard Medical School
Massachusetts Eye and Ear Infirmary
Boston, Massachusetts

Wendy W. Lee, MD, MS (Question 6)
Associate Professor of Clinical Ophthalmology
  & Dermatology
Oculofacial Plastic & Reconstructive Surgery,
  Orbit and Oncology
Bascom Palmer Eye Institute
University of Miami Miller School of Medicine
Miami, Florida

Peter S. Levin, MD (Question 1)
Adjunct Clinical Professor of Ophthalmology
Stanford University
Palo Alto, California

Sophie Liao, MD (Question 42)
Assistant Professor of Ophthalmology
University of Colorado School of Medicine
Aurora, Colorado

Mark J. Lucarelli, MD, FACS (Question 29)
Professor
Director, Oculoplastic, Facial Cosmetic &
  Orbital Surgery
Fellowship in Ophthalmic Facial Plastic Surgery
Madison, Wisconsin

Nicholas R. Mahoney, MD (Question 44)
Assistant Professor of Ophthalmology
Wilmer Eye Institute
Johns Hopkins University
Baltimore, Maryland

Louise A. Mawn, MD, FACS (Question 38)
Associate Professor of Ophthalmology and
  Neurological Surgery
Vanderbilt University Medical Center
Nashville, Tennessee

John D. McCann, MD, PhD (Question 3)
Center for Facial Appearances
Salt Lake City, Utah

Lynda V. McCulley, PharmD (Question 8)
US Food and Drug Administration
Silver Spring, Maryland

Payam V. Morgan, MD (Question 15)
Clinical Instructor
Division of Orbital & Ophthalmic Plastic Surgery
Jules Stein Eye Institute/UCLA
Los Angeles, California

Maryam Nazemzadeh, MD (Question 13)
Fellow, Orbital and Oculofacial Surgery
The Children's Hospital of Philadelphia and
The Edwin and Fannie Gray Hall Center for
    Human Appearance
Perelman School of Medicine
The University of Pennsylvania
Philadelphia, Pennsylvania

Isaac M. Neuhaus, MD (Question 19)
Associate Professor
Department of Dermatology
University of California, San Francisco
San Francisco, California

Danny Ng, FRCS, MPH (Question 46)
Clinical Assistant Professor
Department of Ophthalmology and Visual
    Sciences
The Chinese University of Hong Kong
Hong Kong, China

John Nguyen, MD (Question 33)
Assistant Professor
West Virginia University Eye Institute
Morgantown, West Virginia

Payal Patel, MD (Question 37)
Clinical Instructor of Ophthalmology
NYU Langone Medical Center
New York, New York

Vivek R. Patel, MD (Question 49)
Associate Professor
Director, Neuro-ophthalmology and Adult
    Strabismus
Residency Program Director
USC Eye Institute, Keck School of Medicine
University of Southern California
Los Angeles, California

W. Jordan Piluek, MD (Questions 8, 11)
Wilmer Eye Institute
Johns Hopkins School of Medicine
Baltimore, Maryland

Jerry K. Popham, MD, FACS (Question 7)
Park Avenue Oculoplastic Surgeons, PC
Denver, Colorado

Roxana Rivera, MD (Question 20)
Assistant Professor of Ophthalmology
Division of Oculoplastic and Reconstructive
    Surgery
Wilmer Eye Institute
Johns Hopkins University School of Medicine
Baltimore, Maryland

*Geoffrey E. Rose, BSc, MBBS, MS, DSc, MRCP,
    FRCS, FRCOphth (Question 39)*
Consultant Ophthalmic Surgeon
Adnexal Service, Moorfields Eye Hospital
Honorary Reader in Ophthalmology and
    Senior Research Fellow
NIHR Biomedical Research Centre
UCL Institute of Ophthalmology
Honorary Professor
University of London City University
London, England

Stuart R. Seiff, MD, FACS (Question 36)
Professor of Ophthalmology, Senate Emeritus
University of California San Francisco
Consultant, Orbital and Oculofacial Plastic
    Surgery
California Pacific Medical Center
Mills Peninsula Medical Center
San Francisco, California

Rona Z. Silkiss, MD, FACS (Question 5)
Chief, Division of Oculofacial Plastic Surgery
California Pacific Medical Center
Associate Clinical Professor
University of California, San Francisco
San Francisco, California

Jennifer A. Sivak-Callcott, MD (Question 33)
Professor of Ophthalmology
Director, Ophthalmic Plastic and Reconstructive
    Surgery
West Virginia University Eye Institute
Morgantown, West Virginia

Jonathan Song, MD (Question 40)
Associate Professor of Ophthalmology
USC Eye Institute
USC Keck School of Medicine
Los Angeles, California

Bazil Stoica, MD (Question 47)
Centro Oftalmologico y Oculoplastico de
    Madrid
Hospital de Madrid Norte Sanchinarro
Madrid, Spain

Prem Subramanian, MD, PhD (Question 10)
Professor of Ophthalmology, Neurology, and
    Neurosurgery
Director, Neuro-Ophthalmology
Vice Chair for Academic Affairs, Ophthalmology
University of Colorado School of Medicine
Aurora, Colorado

Timothy J. Sullivan, FRANZCO (Question 32)
Professor of Ophthalmology
Eyelid Lacrimal and Orbital Clinic
Royal Brisbane and Women's Hospital
Brisbane, Australia

Chris Thiagarajah, MD, FACS (Question 9)
Associate Professor of Ophthalmology
Georgetown University Medical Center
Washington, DC

Daniel J. Townsend, MD (Question 14)
Senior Surgeon
Massachusetts Eye and Ear Infirmary
Boston, Massachusetts

David T. Tse, MD, FACS (Question 46)
Vice Chair of Administration and Strategic
    Planning
Professor of Ophthalmology, Dermatology,
    Otolaryngology, and Neurosurgery
Dr. Nasser Ibrahim Al-Rashid Chair in
    Ophthalmic Plastic, Orbital Surgery and
    Oncology
Bascom Palmer Eye Institute
Miami, Florida

Roger E. Turbin, MD (Question 35)
Associate Professor
Institute of Ophthalmology and Visual Sciences,
    Rutgers New Jersey Medical School
Divisions of Neuro-ophthalmology, Orbital and
    Oculoplastic Surgery
Associate Director Neuro-ophthalmology, IOVS
Chief of Neuro-ophthalmology Services
Department of Veterans Affairs Medical Center
East Orange, New Jersey

Ana Carolina Victoria, MD (Question 34)
Oculofacial Plastic and Reconstructive Surgery
Miami, Florida

Timothy S. Wang, MD (Question 23)
Associate Professor
Department of Dermatology
Director
Cutaneous Surgery Unit
Johns Hopkins School of Medicine
Baltimore, MD

Michael T. Yen, MD (Question 27)
Professor of Ophthalmology
Cullen Eye Institute
Baylor College of Medicine
Houston, Texas

Michael K. Yoon, MD (Question 17)
Assistant Professor of Ophthalmology
Harvard Medical School
Massachusetts Eye and Ear Infirmary
Boston, Massachusetts

Siegrid S. Yu, MD (Question 22)
Associate Professor, Department of Dermatology
Director, Procedural Dermatology Fellowship
UCSF Dermatologic Surgery & Laser Center
San Francisco, California

Preface

The informal consult (ie, the curbside consult) is a common and indispensable part of the practice of medicine. The busy clinician faced with a diagnostic or treatment dilemma can solicit practical advice from a knowledgeable expert in a short period of time. Every day across the United States and the world, these brief curbside consultations are taking place in clinic hallways, over the telephone, at lunch, or nowadays by email. The question is typically brief and concise. The advice is practical, to the point, and based on the expert's knowledge, judgment, and experience. It is the essence of the curbside consult that this book wishes to capture.

This volume represents the second edition of *Curbside Consultation in Oculoplastics*. It was developed in response to the enthusiastic acceptance of the first edition and is part of a larger series of textbooks for ophthalmologists by SLACK Incorporated. The goal of the series is to provide a compendium of this type of clinical information: answers to the thorny questions most commonly posed to specialists by residents and practicing colleagues. We hope that this educational question-and-answer–type format will be unique among the available publications in ophthalmology.

We have compiled 49 questions and posed them to master clinicians in the field. In this second edition, some topics are updated and others are entirely new. The clinical advice is based on personal experience but supported by the evidence-based literature. The answers to the curbside questions are designed to meet 4 criteria of content (the 4 Cs): current (timely), concise (summarizing), credible (evidence-based), and clinically relevant (practical).

The primary target audience for this book is the practicing ophthalmologist. We recognize that the management of many of these clinical problems will be controversial, and we emphasize to the reader that the curbside opinions and preferences of the authors represent their viewpoints based on their clinical experience and should not be misinterpreted as a standard of care or a hard and fast rule for every situation.

We hope that you will enjoy reading this book as much as we enjoyed putting it together.

SECTION I

COSMETIC OCULOFACIAL PLASTIC SURGERY

QUESTION

WHAT ARE THE
CURRENT THOUGHTS ON BLEPHAROPLASTY?

Peter S. Levin, MD

How do you minimize the risk for ocular irritation and dry eye after blepharoplasty? How can an unnatural surgical look after blepharoplasty be prevented? Is there ever a role for transcutaneous lower blepharoplasty or should surgery always be performed through a transconjunctival approach? What is the SOOF and how do you lift it? Do you recommend fat repositioning in lower blepharoplasty?

Blepharoplasty is a great procedure and most patients are delighted with their improved appearance and vision. But, every week I see a number of patients in consultation who have had previous blepharoplasty who are not happy, usually for two (often overlapping) reasons. The first is aesthetic disappointment, generally from a hollow, prematurely aged appearance of the upper eyelids or from rounding or retraction of the lower eyelids. The second is that their eyes are irritated after blepharoplasty despite medical management (trials of artificial tears, plugs, and cyclosporine eye drops). In some patients, the irritation is caused by poor closure of the upper lids or retraction of the lower eyelids, but in many patients, the eyelid closure appears complete yet the patient has eyes that are dry and irritated.

Although the mainstay of blepharoplasty surgery remains the removal of excess skin, muscle, and/or fat (so-called subtractive blepharoplasty), the current era of blepharoplasty has improved aesthetics and vision while minimizing the risk for ocular surface problems by minimizing orbicularis oculi excision and preserving periorbital volume by only selectively excising eyelid fat. Recall that the circular orbicularis oculi muscle is responsible for closure of the eyelids. Preserving the orbicularis oculi not only helps to achieve a fuller, more youthful look, but also seems to protect against the development of lagophthalmos. Preservation or repositioning of fat is also thought to achieve a more natural, youthful appearance in selected patients. The eyelids are part of the whole fullness and position of the forehead and midface, and are important considerations to the blepharoplasty surgeon today.

Kersten RC, McCulley TJ, eds. *Curbside Consultation in Oculoplastics:*
49 Clinical Questions, Second Edition (pp 3-8).
© 2016 Taylor & Francis Group.

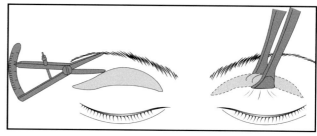

Figure 1-1. Determination of the amount of skin to be excised can be done by either measuring the amount of skin to remain (right eye) or by a pinch test (left eye).

Many patients requesting blepharoplasty have mild symptoms and signs of dry eye syndrome that might relate to such factors as previous LASIK, meibomian gland dysfunction, or aqueous insufficiency. How can we help these patients with surgery, yet avoid the creation or exacerbation of dry eyes and ocular irritation? In my opinion, even patients who are not bothered enough by their symptoms to comply with previously recommended dry eye or external disease therapy should be tuned up prior to blepharoplasty. Among the many possible therapeutic options are frequent artificial tear administration, punctal plugs, prescription of topical or systemic medications in the tetracycline family, topical cyclosporine, warm compresses, and commercial lid scrubs. I tell patients that once surgery is complete and we know that they are doing well without dry eye symptoms, these treatments for dry eyes can be curtailed. Dry eye patients are also educated to expect a conservative result from surgery, which is also in keeping with current trends on aesthetics.

Upper Blepharoplasty Technique

I use techniques that minimize disruption of the normal eyelid blink consisting of conservative skin excision, preservation of all (or most) of the orbicularis oculi muscle, and conservative removal of fat (where indicated) to achieve optimal cosmetic sculpting. The upper blepharoplasty is marked, generally using the patient's existing lid crease and with a conservative upper limb of the ellipse to ensure that skin deficiency is not contributory to the problems of closure. The amount of excised skin can be determined by leaving 10 to 15 mm of skin between the brow and upper limb of the incision, or by the pinch test—avoiding eyelash eversion when the upper and lower limbs of the proposed incision are brought together (Figure 1-1).

A skin-only ellipse is removed initially, leaving the underlying orbicularis undisturbed. This maneuver alone is sometimes adequate to give a pleasing functional and aesthetic result. If additional upper eyelid sculpting is desired, the eyelid can be debulked by removing fat. The medial (frequently removed) and/or central (rarely removed) fat pads of the eyelid are exposed by making small horizontal buttonhole incisions in, and spreading through, the orbicularis muscle. Fat can then be excised using the surgeon's preferred method of fat excision (Figure 1-2). If the eyelid crease is ill defined, then a bit of thermal cautery to the superior border of the tarsus, or excision of a narrow 2-mm strip of orbicularis above the superior tarsal border with fixation of the inferior skin edge to the expansion of the levator aponeurosis, may be useful (Figure 1-3). I like to close the incision with running 6-0 polypropylene suture.

Lower Blepharoplasty Technique

Surgery on the lower eyelid can improve bulging fat and also improve congenital and acquired grooves between the eyelid and cheek. Surgery on the lower eyelid must always avoid lower eyelid

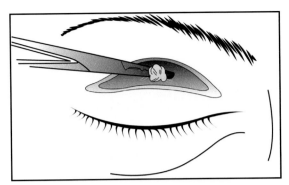

Figure 1-2. Traditionally, fat has been excised with the use of a hemostat followed by excision of fat with scissors. The cut edge of fat is cauterized. Some surgeons prefer to excise fat with a unipolar cautery unit and others with a laser. Meticulous hemostasis is critical.

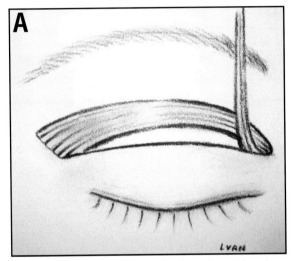
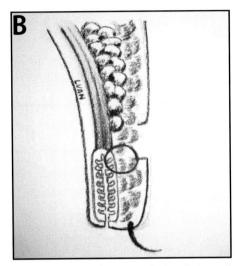

Figure 1-3. The eyelid crease can be given better definition by excision of a small strip of orbicularis oculi muscle (A) exposing the underlying tarsus and levator aponeurosis (B), to which the skin can be secured. (Reprinted with permission from Lynda McCulley, PharmD.)

retraction, while maintaining normal blinking, smiling, and expression. Orbicularis preservation techniques help to achieve these results. Transconjunctival fat excision is a fast and time-honored procedure with minimal risks of exacerbating dry eye problems. I also like to educate patients about current techniques of lower eyelid surgery by lower fat repositioning and suborbicularis oculi fat (SOOF) suspension that have allowed us to improve our aesthetic outcomes with similar levels of safety (Figure 1-4).

Lower eyelid blepharoplasty should be customized to the individual patient's needs. Therefore, it is impossible to describe a single best technique that can be used for all patients. What I will do is describe a lower eyelid blepharoplasty with fat repositioning and orbicularis oculi muscle suspension. This is the procedure that I find appropriate for the majority of patients. It has the potential to fill in a deflated tear trough, as well as reduce baggy eyelids.

The lower eyelid incision is made across the conjunctiva. Dissection proceeds to the inferior orbital rim between the orbicularis and orbital septum. I find a cautery unit or CO_2 laser helpful for this part of the dissection. Dissection then proceeds 10 to 15 mm inferior to the orbital rim in the SOOF, which lies between the orbicularis muscle and the periosteum below. Medially, this dissection lifts the orbicularis from its bony insertion medially at the tear trough (or nasojugal groove). Laterally, the dissection releases the orbicularis retaining ligament, which suspends the orbicularis to the underlying bone (Figure 1-5A).

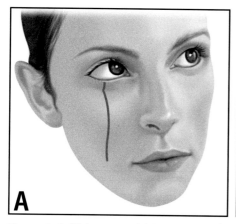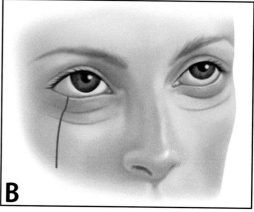

Figure 1-4. (A) Lower eyelid blepharoplasty is aimed at creating a more youthful contour of the lower eyelid and upper cheek. (B) Repositioning of orbital fat or elevation of the midface can be used to reduce the hollow lying between the eyelid and the cheek seen in the aged face.

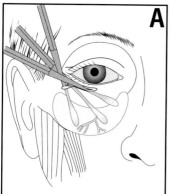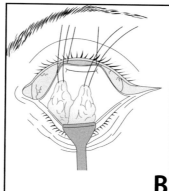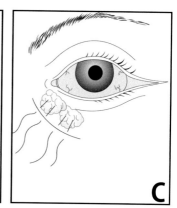

Figure 1-5. (A) Fat repositioning is achieved by dissecting through the suborbicularis oculi fat. (B and C) This creates a pocket in which the orbital fat is secured.

With the lower eyelid retracted inferiorly, the orbital septum is excised, and the medial and central fat pads are pushed into the pocket that is created over the midface. They are then secured into position with horizontal mattress sutures that are brought through the skin of the midface (Figure 1-5B). These are left for several days postoperatively. In a more traditional blepharoplasty, fat would be excised rather than repositioned. These procedures are not mutually exclusive. If there truly is excessive fat, some can be excised and some repositioned.

Next, the orbicularis hammock is tightened. A 15-mm incision is made across the lateral lower eyelid and extended in a laugh line into the lateral canthus. The skin is undermined from orbicularis for 1 cm inferiorly. The orbicularis is cut across the incision and then undermined until the previously dissected suborbicularis pocket is encountered. Additional blunt or sharp dissection may be performed depending on the tension desired on the cheek. The flap of orbicularis muscle is sewn to lateral periosteum with a buried mattress suture of 5-0 chromic. Any excess muscle is trimmed (Figure 1-6).

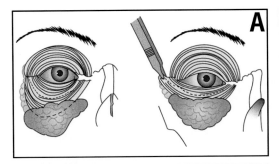

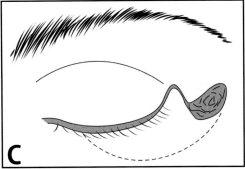

Figure 1-6. (A) Securing the orbicularis oculi hammock is achieved by suspending the lateral orbicularis from the lateral orbital rim. (B) Skin and orbicularis are divided, (C) allowing for the orbicularis muscle to be sutured to the lateral orbital rim, in part independent of the overlying skin.

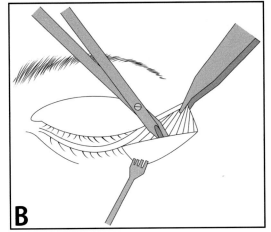

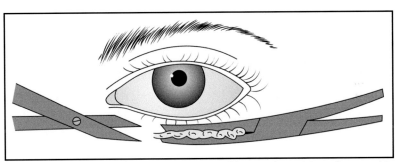

Figure 1-7. Dermatochalasis can be addressed by simple excision of excess skin following crush with a hemostat.

If there is excessive lower eyelid skin, the lower eyelid skin can be pinched with a hemostat (leaving the underlying orbicularis muscle alone) and excised with scissors (Figure 1-7). I like to close the incisions with 6-0 polypropylene.

Current blepharoplasty surgery is aimed at sculpting the upper and lower eyelids with avoidance of lagophthalmos and preservation of orbicularis muscle. Upper blepharoplasty is performed with conservative skin removal, relative preservation of orbicularis oculi muscle, with excision of fat (when indicated) to achieve the desired contour of the upper eyelid. Lower blepharoplasty focuses on fat repositioning or removal, blunting the transition between the lower eyelid and the cheek. Elevation of the SOOF and cheek, in many cases, may also be performed to achieve the desired youthful lower eyelid contour.

Bibliography

Haddock NT, Saadeh PB, Boutros S, Thorne CH. The tear trough and lid/cheek junction: anatomy and implications for surgical correction. *Plast Reconstr Surg.* 2009;123(4):1332-1340.

Hamawy AH, Farkas JP, Fagien S, Rohrich RJ. Preventing and managing dry eyes after periorbital surgery: a retrospective review. *Plast Reconstr Surg.* 2009;123(1):353-359.

Loeb R. *Aesthetic Surgery of the Eyelids.* New York: Springer-Verlag; 1989.

McCord CD Jr, Codner MA, Hester TR. Redraping the inferior orbicularis arc. *Plast Reconstr Surg.* 1998;102(7):2471-2479.

Rohrich RJ, Coberly DM, Fagien S, Stuzin JM. Current concepts in aesthetic upper blepharoplasty. *Plast Reconstr Surg.* 2004;113(3):32e-42e.

Saadat D, Dresner SC. Safety of blepharoplasty in patients with preoperative dry eyes. *Arch Facial Plast Surg.* 2004;6(2):101-104.

Schiller JD. Lysis of the orbicularis retaining ligament and orbicularis oculi insertion: a powerful modality for lower eyelid and cheek rejuvenation. *Plast Reconstr Surg.* 2012;129:692(e)-700(e).

How Can I Address Midface Descent and Volume Depletion?

Roger A. Dailey, MD, FACS

What is the role of the midfacial tissues in supporting the lower eyelid? What can be done to address aging changes of the midface at the time of lower blepharoplasty?

Patients who need or request improvement of the periocular region may benefit from surgery to address volume depletion and descent of the midface. Although these changes can occur for a variety of reasons, the focus of this discussion will be on involution midface changes. A complete understanding of the involved anatomy will then allow the surgeon to choose from myriad treatment possibilities. The importance of an informed patient with realistic expectations in achieving a successful outcome should not be underestimated.

The two main factors that occur with aging of the facial soft tissues are descent and deflation. Descent has long been considered the main factor in aging. Many surgeries have been described to lift the face. More recently, surgeons have come to understand that loss of volume occurs with aging. This too should be addressed to achieve better aesthetic and functional results. Indications for surgical repair include cosmetic correction of midface volume loss relative to the lower face, lower eyelid retraction or ectropion (especially cicatricial), and facial muscle weakness with paralytic ectropion and midface descent.

Correction of Midface Descent

The midface extends from the lower eyelid margin to the inferior aspect of the cheek at about the level of the nasolabial angle. The basic anatomy of this area is shown in Figure 2-1. The subcutaneous fat overlying the malar eminence is referred to as the suborbicularis oculi fat pad (SOOF).[1,2] The surgical approaches to the midface (prezygomatic area) are shown in Figure 2-2.

Kersten RC, McCulley TJ, eds. *Curbside Consultation in Oculoplastics: 49 Clinical Questions, Second Edition* (pp 9-13).
© 2016 Taylor & Francis Group.

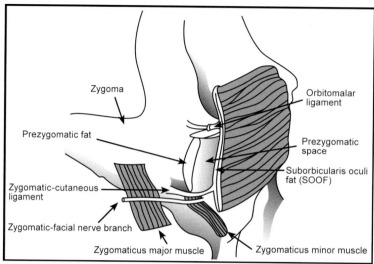

Figure 2-1. Generalized anatomy of the midface region. Make particular note of the orbitomalar ligament, zygomatic-cutaneous ligament, and the SOOF.

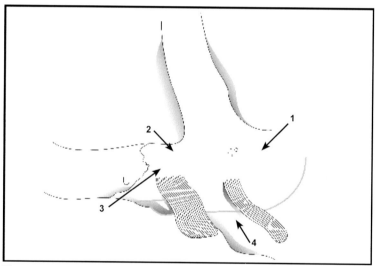

Figure 2-2. The midface (prezygomatic area) can be approached from 4 different routes: (1) superiorly via a transconjunctival inferior fornix incision, (2) temporally via the temporalis fossa, (3) inferotemporally concurrent with a SMAS facelift procedure, or (4) inferiorly via an intraoral mucosa incision in the superior gingival sulcus.

This area can be approached from 4 different routes: (1) superiorly via a transconjunctival inferior fornix incision, (2) temporally via the temporalis fossa, (3) inferotemporally concurrent with a superficial musculoaponeurotic system (SMAS) facelift procedure, or (4) inferiorly via an intraoral mucosa incision in the superior gingival sulcus.[3]

In general, the more midface elevation and volume needed, the more extensive the procedure. The SOOF often descends with aging and can lead to a visible soft tissue depression over the inferior orbital rim, which is referred to as a *tear trough deformity* (Figure 2-3). This often needs to be addressed at the time of lower blepharoplasty, which can be combined with midface lifting.

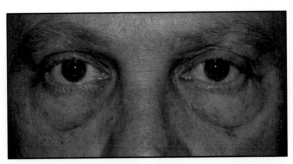

Figure 2-3. Typical appearance of a tear trough deformity associated with fat herniation and midface descent.

In aesthetic patients requiring mild elevation and volume, a lateral canthal incision with swinging lower eyelid flap approach can be used. The soft tissues of the midface are supported by attachments to the underlying periosteum along the infra-orbital rim by two ligamentous attachments known as the orbitomalar and zygomatic-cutaneous ligaments. Preperiosteal dissection over the face of the maxilla results in release of these attachments, which then allows adequate mobility of the SOOF. Two 3-0 monocryl sutures are then used to anchor the SOOF to the intermediate temporalis fascia just above the zygomatic arch and periosteum overlying the zygoma. Excess orbicularis can be resected and then further suspended to the periosteum with absorbable suture laterally (Figures 2-4 through 2-7).

In cases where a more robust elevation is desired, the prezygomatic area can be reached via a subconjunctival incision, a temporal brow incision, and even an intraoral incision. The temporal brow incision allows elevation of the upper lateral face so that a standing wave does not occur at the lateral canthus due to excessive elevation of the midface relative to lax temporal scalp. The temporal dissection occurs in the subtemporoparietal plane just above the deep temporalis fascia and then enters the midface in a subperiosteal plane.[4] A transconjunctival incision is added if a lower lid fat transposition over the rim is going to be done in conjunction, or a posterior lamellar graft such as Enduragen, Alloderm, or autogenous hard palate graft is going to be placed. A lateral canthal incision can be added if a lower lid blepharoplasty requiring lid shortening and skin or muscle resection is going to be done concurrently. The intraoral incision can facilitate the placement of periosteal cheek sutures for suspension, but is not necessary.

In certain patients who are particularly short of anterior lamellar skin, in need of some midface volume, or unlikely to have good supporting tissue for some reason (eg, aged older than 60 years, poor protoplasm, or connective tissue disease), a hand-carved, expanded polytetrafluoroethylene orbital rim implant can be placed.[5] The advantage of this, in addition to providing volume, is that the sutures can be placed from the SOOF to the Goretex (W. L. Gore and Associates Inc) along the entire superior midface to give excellent and lasting vertical lift of the central and nasal midface. The implant should be rigidly fixed to the rim prior to attaching the soft tissues of the midface with self-drilling screws (Figure 2-8).

Correction of Volume Depletion

Techniques for volume restoration include fillers, fat grafting, surgical elevation of soft tissues into the midface, and placement of midface implants. Volume enhancement via surgery, with or without cheek implants, has already been discussed. Fillers are commonly used in the midface. Previously, it was a reasonable idea to start off with a hyaluronic acid filler such as Restylane or

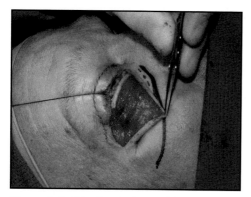

Figure 2-4. Skin flap is elevated from infraciliary crease.

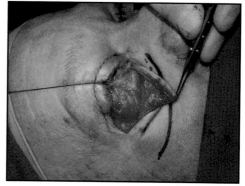

Figure 2-5. The orbital fat is accessed via a transconjunctival-swinging lower eyelid flap that contains the orbital septum and orbicularis muscle.

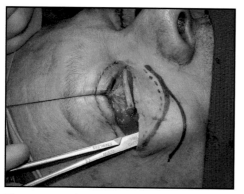

Figure 2-6. The scissors are being used to release the orbitomalar ligament and the zygomatic-cutaneous ligaments prior to supraperiosteal midface elevation.

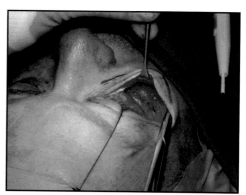

Figure 2-7. Supraperiosteal dissection view from superiorly.

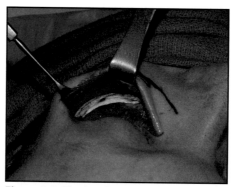

Figure 2-8. The hand-carved Goretex block is rigidly fixed just below the orbital rim and is ready for sutures to be placed from the SOOF to the Goretex to provide excellent and lasting vertical lift.

Juvéderm to ensure the patient had midfacial volume improvement and tolerated the product well. If not, hyaluronidase could be injected into the filled area and resolve any unwanted effects, usually within a few hours. Once it was clear that the fill was appreciated, a longer-lasting filler such as Perlane, Radiesse, or Sculptra could be used.[6] With the recent FDA approval of Juvéderm Voluma, marked improvement of volume depletion and even some midface descent can be managed with this filler.[7] This may reduce the number of patients needing surgery. In cases of significant descent, Voluma should be a welcome addition to the management arsenal, reducing the need for implants and more extensive surgery and allowing for a natural and pleasing final aesthetic and functional result. In general, fillers in the midface should be placed just superficial to the periosteum in the upper midface and certainly deep to the orbicularis initially to avoid lumpiness. Postinjection massage by the injector is important to obtain a smooth result. In patients with reasonably thick skin, Restylane can be used more superficially in the tear trough if placed by an experienced injector. Certain anatomic structures such as the lacrimal sac, facial nerve, and parotid duct should be avoided. I find antegrade injection to be helpful here and it may be safer because it pushes blood vessels out of the way, lessening the chance of intravascular injection, which may produce tissue necrosis and loss leading to scarring. Blindness has also been reported, so in addition to antegrade injection, one should consider lower pressure and smaller aliquots in this and other risky areas such as the glabella and alar base area.

Autogenous fat injections can also be used to create volume in the midface.[8] Once the fat is harvested by liposuction techniques from the surgeon's area of choice, it is injected into the deep tissues of the midface below the orbicularis in a fan-like fashion. If the lower eyelid is to be included, the approach should be performed in such a way that the tunnels made by the injection cannula are oriented vertically and not horizontally to avoid a sausage roll appearance in the lid. For further information about fillers, see Question 5.

Summary

Aging and functional changes of the midface that involve descent and depletion can be corrected by several different surgical interventions to reposition the tissues anatomically into a more youthful and functional position and provide appropriate volume. Further volume can be added with cheek implants, fillers, or autogenous fat.

References

1. Kikkawa DO, Lemke BN, Dortzbach RK. Relations of the superficial musculoaponeurotic system to the orbit and characterization of the orbitomalar ligament. *Ophthal Plast Reconstr Surg*. 1996;12(2):77-88.
2. Lucarelli MJ, Khwarg SI, Lemke BN, Kozel JS, Dortzbach RK. The anatomy of midface ptosis. *Ophthal Plast Reconstr Surg*. 2000;16(1):7-22.
3. Mendelson BC, Muzaffar AR, Adams WP. Surgical anatomy of the midcheek and malar mounds. *Plast Reconstr Surg*. 2002;110(3):885-896.
4. Sullivan SA, Dailey RA. Endoscopic subperiosteal midface lift. *Ophthal Plast Reconstr Surg*. 2002;18(5):319-330.
5. Steinsapir KD. Aesthetic and restorative midface lifting with hand-carved, expanded polytetrafluoroethylene orbital rim implants. *Plast Reconstr Surg*. 2003;111(5):1727-1737.
6. O'Hara KL, Urrego AF, Garri JI, O'Hara CM, Bradley JP, Kawamoto HK. Improved malar projection with transconjunctival hydroxyapatite granules. *Plast Reconstr Surg*. 2006;117(6):1956-1963.
7. Callan P, Goodman GJ, Carlisle I, et al. Efficacy and safety of a hyaluronic acid filler in subjects treated for correction of midface volume deficiency: a 24 month study. *Clin Cosmet Investig Dermatol*. 2013;6:81-89.
8. Pontius AT, Williams EF. The evolution of midface rejuvenation. Combining the midface-lift and fat transfer. *Arch Facial Plast Surg*. 2006;8:300-305.

WHAT IS THE CURRENT SURGICAL APPROACH FOR BROW PTOSIS REPAIR?

Robert C. Kersten, MD, FACS and
John D. McCann, MD, PhD

A 55-year-old male presents with complaints of the upper eyelids blocking his vision to the point where he has to raise his brows constantly to see. He is also concerned with his tired facial appearance and the heaviness of the upper eyelids (Figure 3-1). He would like something done to improve his vision as well as his facial appearance. A visual field test showed obscuration of greater than 50% of the superior visual field. This reverted to normal with mechanical elevation of the eyelids. What should be done to treat his condition?

Eyebrow ptosis is an important and frequent functional as well as cosmetic diagnosis in oculoplastic surgery. As the eyelids lose elasticity with gravity and aging, so do the forehead and eyebrows. It is common for a patient to have dermatochalasis, eyelid ptosis, and brow ptosis simultaneously. When a patient has excess tissue and heaviness in the upper eyelids, it is important that the position of the eyebrows is also evaluated and the proposed intervention address the totality of upper facial malposition.

A common mistake of eye surgeons is failing to recognize the brow ptosis component when evaluating patients with dermatochalasis, ptosis, and fat prolapse in the upper eyelids. Blepharoplasty and eyelid ptosis repair performed alone in the presence of significant brow ptosis can result in further lowering of brow position with negative functional and cosmetic consequences. The separation between the eyelid margin and the brow is reduced and patients may develop lagophthalmos that may require skin grafting.

When marked brow ptosis is present, an upper blepharoplasty and ptosis repair without brow elevation or stabilization may result in worsening of brow ptosis when the visual axis is cleared, because reflexive recruitment of the frontalis to elevate the eyelid is no longer required. Excision of eyelid skin in the presence of significant brow ptosis can also displace the thick skin of the brow

Kersten RC, McCulley TJ, eds. *Curbside Consultation in Oculoplastics:*
49 Clinical Questions, Second Edition (pp 15-22).
© 2016 Taylor & Francis Group.

Figure 3-1. Clinical photograph of a 55-year-old male with brow ptosis and dermatochalasis resulting in a tired facial appearance.

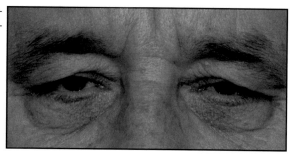

further downward into the upper eyelid, narrowing the space between the eyelashes and the brow hairs, resulting in an undesired angry or concerned appearance.

Diagnosing brow ptosis and having an armamentarium of procedures available to treat it is essential for the eyelid surgeon. The brow is depressed medially by the corrugator and depressor supercilii muscles, which are involved in frowning. The medial orbicularis oculi muscle is also involved to some degree. People who frown frequently develop hypertrophy and hypertonicity of these muscles with resultant downward slanting of the medial brow. Loss of skin elasticity with age makes the problem more overt. This is more common in males, although it is seen in both males and females who spend considerable time outdoors and use the brows to protect their eyes from the sun. Corrugator muscle contraction results in vertical furrow lines in the glabellar region, whereas procerus muscle contraction is responsible for the horizontal lines at the base of the nose. The temporal tail of the eyebrow is also prone to droop over time because the brow elevator frontalis muscle doesn't extend laterally beyond the temporal line, leaving the temporal eyebrow unsupported against gravitational induced dependency.

Dysfunction of the frontalis muscle results in global brow descent. This may occur due to facial nerve dysfunction, either through idiopathic Bell's palsy or trauma to the frontal branch of cranial nerve VII (accidents or surgery), or it may be chemically induced at the myoneural junction (Botulinum toxin). Patients with facial nerve damage have a more profound degree of brow ptosis, and if the zygomatic branch of cranial nerve VII is also involved there will be associated paralysis of the upper and lower eyelid orbicularis, which can result in more severe functional consequences due to lagophthalmos and exposure keratopathy.

Determining the pathophysiology of brow ptosis for each individual patient is essential for achieving the optimal functional as well as cosmetic outcome. Patients presenting with functional complaints may be less concerned with cosmesis, although unsightly scars, a surprised appearance, a masculine appearance of the brows in females, or an effeminizing appearance in males will result in unhappy patients regardless of their initial motivation in seeking surgery. With rare exceptions, patients want cosmetic improvement as much as they want improved visual function.

Two important issues to address in the preoperative evaluation are symmetry and contour. Many patients with asymmetrical brows are not aware of this. It is important to point out the brow asymmetry and give the patient reasonable expectations of what can be done to correct this. Eyebrow asymmetry is typically part of facial asymmetry, with the eyebrow being lower on the smaller side of the face. A great deal of facial asymmetry is caused by asymmetry of the facial bones. Eyebrow and forehead surgery can be expected to reduce, but not completely correct, asymmetry because these surgeries do not address the bone.

Another important issue to address is the desired contour. Some patients have primarily medial brow ptosis, which is often caused by strong medial forehead depressors. In these patients, elevation of the medial brow more than the lateral brow is desirable. Other patients have more descent of the lateral brow, which gives people a sad or tired appearance. These patients require more

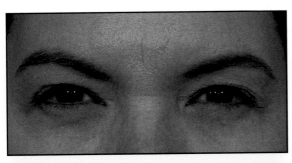

Figure 3-2. Preoperative clinical photograph of a patient who underwent internal brow sculpting with removal of the corrugator and depressor supercilii muscles. Note the marked dermatochalasis and brow ptosis.

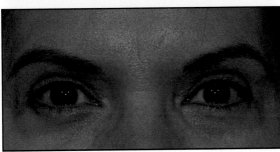

Figure 3-3. Postoperative clinical photograph of patient who underwent internal brow sculpting with removal of the corrugator and depressor supercilii muscles. Note the higher medial, central, and lateral brow position.

lateral elevation. Most women prefer lateral flare to the brows, while most men prefer a fairly flat eyebrow configuration. It is particularly important to avoid over-elevation of the lateral brow in patients who have strong medial depressors to avoid a surprised or quizzical appearance.

Many patients presenting with the complaint of heavy eyelids do not realize that a significant part of their problem is brow ptosis rather than dermatochalasis. Their usual concern is the excess skin on the upper eyelids and/or eyelid droopiness that blocks their superior field of vision, prevents them from wearing makeup, and gives a tired facial appearance. It is the surgeon's responsibility to define the various problems and take the amount of time necessary to explain the treatment modalities required to give the expected functional and cosmetic result.

There are a number of surgical procedures that are in use today for the correction of brow ptosis. Some are more effective, more involved, and more expensive than others and none is perfect for all patients. Historically, these procedures have been grouped as less invasive and more invasive, based on the extent of surgery and recovery involved. The less invasive procedures include internal brow lifting procedures performed through the upper lid blepharoplasty incision site. The more invasive procedures include coronal forehead lifts and the pretrichial brow lift. The endoscopic brow lift is viewed by most patients and physicians as being less invasive because it requires only several short incisions hidden in the scalp.

The internal brow lift involves internal brow sculpting with concomitant reattachment of the brow in a higher position (brow pexy). Although the exact benefit is debated, attaching the brow to the periosteum above the orbital rim is commonly performed by many surgeons today. In some patients, the brow fat is not in excess but has simply prolapsed inferiorly. In these cases, the brow fat is suspended superiorly with sutures.

In our experience, if the medial brow is low, the brow depressor muscles are best myotomized or excised. The corrugator and depressor supercili are weakened or excised while the procerus is disinserted, allowing for reinsertion in the healing phase in a more superior position. Removing the brow depressors allows the frontalis muscle to more effectively elevate the medial and central brow. This procedure is done through the upper eyelid blepharoplasty incision (Figure 3-2). We have found this to be the most effective and permanent modality to elevate the medial brow (Figure 3-3).

Figure 3-4. Preoperative photograph showing marked dermatochalasis and brow ptosis in a patient who underwent an endoscopic brow lift.

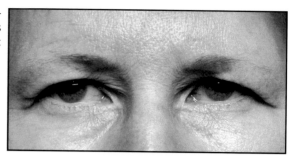

Direct Brow Lift

The direct brow lift has limited application because it tends to heal with visible scars. It is an appropriate procedure in some elderly non-aesthetically motivated patients. The greater abundance of brow hair in males makes the scar easier to camouflage, but the crescent shaped "arched" brow that results after direct skin excision paralleling the eyebrow and tapering at its medial and temporal terminus is more consistent with the normal brow position found in females. The medial brow has thicker, more sebaceous skin, which usually results in a more visible scar than the thinner skin above the lateral brow. The direct brow lift has its greatest application in female patients with facial nerve palsy, which is usually asymmetrical and requires substantial lateral brow elevation. These patients are more accepting of the visible scar because of the marked degree of functional impairment. Patients with symmetrical temporal brow ptosis also are nicely managed with a direct temporal browplasty, as this results in a very effective and predictable elevation of the temporal eyebrow and leaves a largely imperceptible scar.

Mid-Forehead Lift

In male patients with male-pattern baldness or unilateral brow ptosis due to cranial nerve VII paresis who do not want the arched feminized appearance that usually occurs following a full (rather than just lateral) direct browplasty, another acceptable option is the mid-forehead browplasty. Here, an incision is made encompassing one of the transverse forehead rhytids, which allows camouflage of the scar postoperatively. Elliptical excision of an appropriate height of skin—usually about 1 cm—is carried out across the forehead overlying the ptotic eyebrow. Subcutaneous dissection is carried inferiorly over the forehead down to undermine and mobilize the ptotic brow so that it can be supra-placed and anchored to the underlying frontalis muscle with deep sutures to take tension off of the skin incision, which is then closed. This results in dependable and long-lasting elevation of the eyebrow and avoids the crescent surprised, feminized contour that results from a direct, full brow-width incision. In males with transverse forehead rhytids, the scar hidden within the rhytid is barely perceptible (Figure 3-4).

Endoscopic Lift

The endoscopic forehead lift is an elegant way to lift the brows while simultaneously performing a face lift of the upper third of the face. The endoscopic forehead lift elevates the brow to a more youthful position with minimal forehead lengthening, postoperative incision line scarring, or scalp anesthesia. For this reason, it is currently the preferred method for elevating the brows in

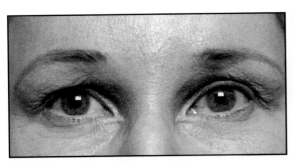

Figure 3-5. Postoperative photograph showing uniformly higher brow position and significant improvement of dermatochalasis in a patient who underwent an endoscopic brow lift.

many aesthetically oriented patients (see Figure 3-4). In addition to brow elevation, it provides a dramatic reduction in forehead furrow lines by accomplishing a subperiostial lift of the upper third of the face. The endoscopic forehead lift also allows for some elevation of the midface and even an improvement in the lateral periocular crow's feet area.

The endoscopic forehead procedure is done through 3 small radial incisions just behind the hairline that allow access to the subperiosteal space between the 2 temporal lines of fusion. This results in great elevation of the central and mid-forehead and brows. Proper elevation of the lateral brow requires an additional temporal incision on each side. The temporal incisions are used to separate the superficial temporalis fascia from the deep temporalis fascia and to release the confluence of fascia along the temporal lines of fusion. The forehead is anchored to the bone via the paracentral incisions using absorbable post and sutures. Laterally, the superficial temporalis fascia is elevated and anchored to the superficial layer of the deep temporalis fascia with resorbable sutures. Some surgeons still use permanent sutures and screws for this procedure, which, in our experience, is not necessary and can lead to postoperative complications. Sutures and screws that last 6 months are sufficient because the periosteum is already reattached to the frontal bone by that time (Figure 3-5).

The endoscopic forehead lift can be combined with an upper eyelid blepharoplasty if the dermatochalasis is not satisfactorily addressed by the forehead lift alone.

In our experience, endoscopic forehead lifting is the most effective technique for elevating the central and lateral brow. However, without removing the depressor muscles medially, the medial brow will not be maximally elevated. For this reason, if the patient has a low medial brow, we now routinely remove the depressor muscles through either an upper eyelid blepharoplasty incision or from above using the endoscopic technique. If the depressor muscles are not removed, they are treated with Botox to weaken them, allowing the central periostium to heal in an elevated position. If the primary goal is to elevate the lateral brow relative to the medial brow, we do not remove the medial depressors because it can result in a flat or downward slanting configuration to the brows.

Pretrichial Browplasty

In patients with a high hairline, elevation of the forehead through either a coronal or endoscopic approach will result in further lengthening of the forehead, which may be cosmetically undesirable. In these cases, a pretrichial incision at the anterior edge of the hairline can be used to elevate the forehead and excise the excessive visible forehead skin. This requires that an incision be made full thickness through the soft tissues to reach the subperiosteal plane of dissection overlying frontal bone and results in severing of the distal branches of the supraorbital nerve, with resultant hypesthesia from that point posteriorly to the vertex of the skull. Sensation usually returns in 9 to 12 months and if patients are warned of this ahead of surgery, it is usually well tolerated. The

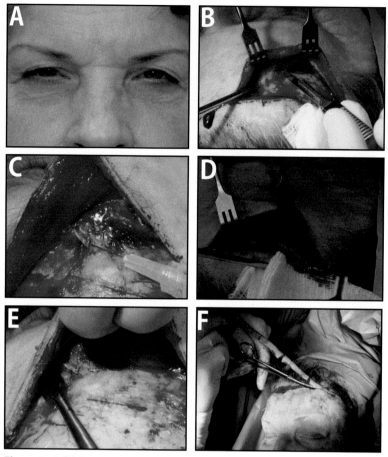

Figure 3-6. (A) Preoperative photograph demonstrating brow ptosis causing superior visual field loss. Once the incision is made, dissection is carried out in the pre-periosteal plane with either (B) a number 10 blade or (C) a blunt finger. (D) The supra-orbital neurovascular bundle is identified and protected as it emerges from the supra-orbital notch or foramen. (E) Once the forehead flap has been released, and the corrugators and procerus debulked, excess soft tissue is estimated by applying superior traction on the flap. (F) The excess is trimmed using "super-sharp" scissors, bevelled slightly superiorly to allow hair follicles to grow up through the undersurface of the flap. (*continued*)

incision heals quite imperceptibly with time but most patients prefer to alter their hair style so that bangs can be combed over the hairline to camouflage the scar.

The results from pretrichial excision of skin tend to be more long-lasting than the repositioning of soft tissues affected by endoscopic lifting where excess frontal skin is redistributed over the scalp (Figure 3-6).

Unfortunately, the treatment of brow ptosis is rarely covered by insurance plans, whether it is affecting vision or not, and many patients reject any procedure that is not covered by insurance. In this instance, it is important that they understand that the best functional and cosmetic result will not be achieved. The cost of the procedure is an important issue whenever a patient is paying for a procedure out of pocket. An advantage of the internal brow lifting procedure is that it can be performed in-office under local anesthesia, compared to an endoscopic forehead lift, which in our experience requires deep sedation or general anesthesia and must be performed in a surgery center.

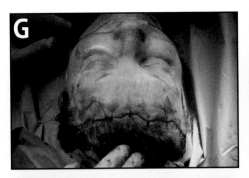
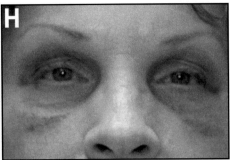
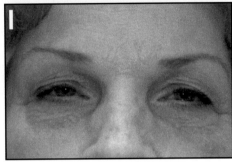

Figure 3-6. (continued) (G) The flap is then opposed to the scalp using horizontal mattress subcutaneous 4-0 vicryl sutures. (H) Staples are then used to approximate the skin across the width of the wound. The exposed pre-trichial skin is then closed with a running 6-0 Prolene suture. The pre-trichial staples are removed after 3 to 4 days while the 6-0 Prolene suture is removed at 1 week. (I) Appearance of postoperative day 4 just prior to staple removal.

Procedures that can be performed in-office give the surgeon greater control over the cost and are inevitably less expensive for the patient. The lower cost and the ability to address brow ptosis using periocular incisions increases patient acceptance of the internal brow lifting procedure, despite the fact that endoscopic forehead lift surgery typically results in a more dramatic improvement.

Summary

Excess eyelid skin, droopy upper eyelids, and droopy eyebrows all tend to occur in the same patient. It is not possible to achieve a good cosmetic and functional result unless all 3 components are addressed. The techniques of correcting eyebrow ptosis that leave the least scarring and give the best cosmetic result include internal brow elevation, endoscopic forehead lift, and corrugator resection. In patients with a long forehead, pretrichial excision of the scalp or mid-forehead excision gives long-term correction of eyebrow elevation but involves a finely visible scar, and in the case of pretrichial excision, temporary hypesthesia of the scalp. These modern techniques are typically not covered by insurance companies, so proper patient counseling is paramount so that patient expectations can be met.

Suggested Readings

Booth AJ, Murray A, Tyers AG. The direct brow lift: efficacy, complications, and patient satisfaction. *Br J Ophthalmol.* 2004;88(5):688-691.

Burroughs JR, Bearden WH, Anderson RL, McCann JD. Internal brow elevation at blepharoplasty. *Arch Facial Plast Surg.* 2006;8(1):36-41.

Cook BE Jr, Lucarelli MJ, Lemke BN. Depressor supercilii muscle: anatomy, histology, and cosmetic implications. *Ophthal Plast Reconstr Surg.* 2001;17(6):404.

Knize DM. An anatomically based study of the mechanism of eyebrow ptosis. *Plast Reconstr Surg.* 1996;97(7):1321-1333.

Pedroza F, dos Anjos GC, Bedoya M, Rivera M. Update on brow and forehead lifting. *Curr Opin Otolaryngol Head Neck Surg.* 2006;14(4):283-288.

Presti P, Yalamanchili H, Honrado CP. Rejuvenation of the aging upper third of the face. *Facial Plast Surg.* 2006;22(2):91-96.

Ramirez OM. Endoscopically assisted biplanar forehead lift. *Plast Reconstr Surg.* 1995;96(2):323-333.

Tyers AG. Brow lift via the direct and trans-blepharoplasty approaches. *Orbit.* 2006;25(4):261-265. Review.

Walden JL, Orseck MJ, Aston SJ. Current methods for brow fixation: are they safe? *Aesthetic Plast Surg.* 2006;30(5):541-548.

WHAT ARE YOUR RECOMMENDATIONS REGARDING ASIAN BLEPHAROPLASTY?

William Chen, MD

How do you approach eyelid surgery in Asian patients? What are the specific qualities that need to be considered when creating an eyelid crease? What complications are most common with cosmetic eyelid crease manipulation?

In Asian blepharoplasty, the goal is to add or enhance an incomplete eyelid crease. The basic need is to create a natural crease appropriate to the ethnic background of your client, which may be approached in 2 ways:

1. An abbreviated non–tissue-removing technique (ie, suture method, nonincisional method, minimal incision methods): Trans-lid compressive sutures are placed to effect a crease indentation. The crease formed this way is from compressive ligation of the skin, orbicularis, levator aponeurosis, and Müller's muscle.

2. The external incision method: A crease that is constructed through removal of some excess skin, soft tissues (fat and excess orbicularis oculi), followed by placement of crease-forming sutures between eyelid skin and aponeuroses that are then completely removed after 7 days, effecting a dynamic crease (which fades when the patient's lid is turned down).

Each technique has its fervent proponents. I favor the external incision method[1] because it can better achieve the following benchmarks:

- Control of the shape of the crease
- Height of the crease
- Continuity of the crease formed
- Permanence of the crease

Kersten RC, McCulley TJ, eds. *Curbside Consultation in Oculoplastics:*
49 Clinical Questions, Second Edition (pp 23-26).
© 2016 Taylor & Francis Group.

Avoidance of Complications

The most frequently encountered complication is asymmetry of the creases of the two eyelids, which may involve the height and/or the shape.

In the suture method, despite its reported simplicity, success requires seasoned practice to achieve symmetrical results. Its greatest challenge is that for individuals with even slight asymmetry in palpebral fissure size, the creation of a resultant crease on each side that looks similar may require the physician to apply the trans-lid sutures from a slightly different position on each side of the eyelid, whether from the conjunctival side or the skin side. The crease looks fine in the short term, although after several years it may induce a Faden effect (weakening of the levator lift) in a differential manner in each eyelid, which may result in asymmetric ptosis. The suture method may also result in fading of crease indentation as the buried suture relaxes its compressive ligation of the soft tissue. This especially limits its utility in patients with significant fat in the upper eyelid. It can also result in the appearance of a dimpled area on the skin where the sutures are buried, as well as a foreign body sensation on the lids.

In external incision methods, the possible complications are similar to those seen with any aesthetic upper blepharoplasty. Attention to where the incisions are made, tissue handling technique, control of bleeding, careful placement of crease-forming sutures, and design of the shape and height will eliminate most of the complications seen with a basic upper blepharoplasty.

Preoperative Anatomy

It is important to observe, photo-document, and share your preoperative findings with your patients. This may include the eyelid fissure's horizontal dimension, height of the opening of the eyelids, levator excursion measurement, range of motion of the extraocular muscles (particularly superior rectus muscle impairment), and presence or absence of Bell's protective reflex. If ptosis is present, it is best repaired first before any attempt is made to create a lid crease.

Counseling

Preoperative counseling is essential to ensure an optimal outcome—not just anatomically but also psychologically and emotionally. I find it advantageous to simulate the crease form in the office using a paperclip wire or a thin-gauged lacrimal probe. I also encourage patients to try it at home so that they become familiar with the look they can expect after the procedure. The usual precaution is given regarding cessation of blood thinning drugs like aspirin, ibuprofen, naproxen, and Coumadin. It is also advised to discontinue fish oil and vitamin E.

It is quite common that patients expect instant recovery, which is unrealistic. I advise patients that the upper eyelids move more than 10,000 times a day and so they cannot expect the area to heal in a week.

Counseling for lid crease revision cases is more extensive and will include a different set of expectations, with a higher rate of uncertainty and lower expectations compared to that of Asian blepharoplasty patients. The success of the outcome has to be measured against the patient's current state and not against a pristine unoperated anatomy. Very detailed photographic documentation of the crease, scarring, and lid anatomy in every angle and macro close-up is taken so that the patient can clearly see and understand his or her preoperative issues. These also serve for comparison in case the patient forgets what his or her problems were. I do not operate on patients for revision unless I feel I can substantially help them improve, and therefore there are cases that I decline.

The Trapezoidal Approach in Asian Blepharoplasty

It is beyond the scope of this brief chapter to cover the entire subject. However, the basic steps are the following:

1. Marking of the crease shape and height based on tarsal height and the patient's request (assessed by the practitioner)

2. Skin incision

3. Transaction through the orbicularis superiorly in a beveled approach

4. Opening of the orbital septum

5. Treatment and preservation of the fat pad (may involve releasing, partial trimming, repositioning). Although the pretarsal fat is usually removed, it is imperative that the preaponeurotic fat be maintained. A deep superior sulcus is undesirable in an Asian eyelid.

6. Trimming of the skin-orbicularis muscle strip along the superior tarsal border

7. Resetting the tissue plane

8. Wound closure with crease construction

Postoperative Management

Patients apply ice compresses to the upper eyelids and are instructed to continue icing as well as bed rest for 1 day. Patients may bathe and sit up for meals the first day; they are told to have restricted physical exertion the first week. Topical gentamicin-steroid ointment (Pred-G, Allergan) is applied 4 times daily for 1 week. Suture removal is usually in 1 week. Patients are told that 80% of swelling should subside within 2 weeks. The crease is not judged until about 3 months out.

My concept of trapezoidal debulking of preaponeurotic platform as applied to Asian blepharoplasty offers the following advantages:

- Accurate preoperative definition of the desired crease height and shape.

- A controlled, layered, and selective treatment of each eyelid's specific findings.

- Atraumatic dissection, precise hemostasis, and prevention of tissue injury, which reduce intraoperative soft tissue distortion and afford more accurate results. This establishes the proper orientation and spatial geometry of the semi-rigid pretarsal skin and tarsus (posterior lamella, vectored by the levator muscle) relative to the more passive preseptal skin and orbicularis (anterior lamella) when the lids are opened.

- Preservation of the preaponeurotic adipose tissue is key in preserving an Asian appearance to the upper eyelid and preventing a sunken superior sulcus.

- Resetting the eyelid skin and forehead structures relative to the posterior lamella prevents the distortion of the skin-levator-skin closure and the resultant crease that is formed.

- Exact anastomosis of levator aponeurosis to lid crease incision along the superior tarsal border ensures a natural crease that is dynamic and disappears on downward gaze as opposed to the skin-tarsus-skin technique (static lid crease).

Reference

1. Chen W. Concept of triangular, trapezoidal and rectangular debulking of eyelid tissues: application in Asian blepharoplasty. *Plast Reconstr Surg.* 1996;97(1):212-218.

Suggested Readings

Chen WPD. Beveled approach for revisional surgery in Asian blepharoplasty. *Plast Reconstr Surg.* 2007;120(2):545-552.
Chen WPD. The concept of a glide zone as it relates to upper lid crease, lid fold, and application in upper blepharoplasty. *Plast Reconstr Surg.* 2007;119(1):379-386.
Chen WPD. *Asian Blepharoplasty and the Eyelid Crease.* 3rd ed. Philadelphia, PA: Elsevier: 2015.
Chen WPD, Khan J. *Color Atlas of Cosmetic Oculofacial Surgery.* Saunders/Elsevier Science, Ltd; 2010.

QUESTION

WHAT IS YOUR FAVORITE FILLER AND WHY?

Rona Z. Silkiss, MD, FACS

I've been hearing a lot about fillers. What role do they play in your oculoplastics practice? How do I choose the best type for my patient?

In the world of fillers, one size does not fit all. An optimal outcome can be achieved by pairing the patient's anatomic changes and desired results with the filler best suited to meet those needs. The selection of the optimal filler may be difficult because there are so many fillers to choose from, many of which differ minimally from their competitor products. This chapter will present an overview of the current fillers available for use in the United States, with commentary as to their optimal use.

Fillers may be used to improve an isolated fold or depression or elevate a wrinkle. They may also be used to provide global facial volumization and reinflation. There are different fillers for each purpose. The choice of filler is determined by exploiting the molecular qualities of the filler with the anatomic changes and rejuvenative requests of the patient. Table 5-1 details many of the current fillers available for use.

The hyaluronic acid–based fillers (hyalurons) are the workhorse fillers for isolated fold or depression improvement. Restylane, Perlane, Juvéderm and their lidocaine-incorporated equivalents (Restylane-L, Perlane-L, Juvéderm XC) are composed of hyaluronic acid manufactured in the lab with streptococci. This is a naturally occurring glycosaminoglycan polymer. The different hyaluron products have varying viscosity and longevity based on the percentage of cross-linked hyaluron, the density of the molecules, and particle size. Only the cross-linked hyaluron resists free radical oxidative and enzymatic degradation, leading to increased longevity in the body.

These fillers do not require skin testing. They can be dissolved with hyaluronidase (Hylenex, Vitrase) in the event of a contour asymmetry or overcorrection. Additionally, these agents induce some collagen synthesis in the area of injection, augmenting their longevity.

Kersten RC, McCulley TJ, eds. *Curbside Consultation in Oculoplastics:*
49 Clinical Questions, Second Edition (pp 27-32).
© 2016 Taylor & Francis Group.

Table 5-1
Fillers, Composition, and Indications for Use

Filler	Composition	Manufacturer Indications
Restylane	Hyaluronic acid 20 mg/mL Cross linked 16 mg/mL Bacterial fermentation	Medicis FDA approval 2003 Fine to medium rhytids
Restylane L	Hyaluronic acid 20 mg/mL Cross linked 16 mg/mL Bacterial fermentation	Medicis FDA approval 2010 Fine to medium rhytids
Perlane	Hyaluronic acid 24 mg/mL Bacterial fermentation	Medicis FDA approval 2007 Medium to deep rhytids
Perlane L	Hyaluronic acid 24 mg/mL Bacterial fermentation Lidocaine 0.3%	Medicis FDA approval 2010 Medium to deep rhytids
Juvéderm	Hyaluronic acid 24 mg/mL Cross linked HA 21.6 mg/mL Bacterial fermentation	Allergan FDA approval 2006 Fine to medium rhytids
Juvéderm Ultra XC	Hyaluronic acid 24 mg/mL Bacterial fermentation Lidocaine 0.3%	Allergan FDA approval 2006 Medium to deep rhytids
Juvéderm Ultra Plus XC	Hyaluronic acid 24 mg/mL Bacterial fermentation Lidocaine 0.3%	Allergan FDA approval 2006 Medium to deep rhytids
Belotero	Hyaluronic acid 22.5 mg/mL	Merz FDA approval 2011 Fine rhytids
Juvéderm Voluma XC	Hyaluronic acid, 20 mg/mL Lidocaine 0.3% Vycross technology	Allergan FDA approval 2013 Midface augmentation
Radiesse	Calcium hydroxyl apatite Can dilute with lidocaine	Biofirm FDA approval 2006 Deep rhytids or folds
Sculptra	Poly-L-lactic acid	Sanofi-Aventis FDA approval 2009 Facial volumization, lipoatrophy

Radiesse, or calcium hydroxyl apatite, is a thicker, more long-lasting filler. It may induce collagenesis in the area of fill. Radiesse is not easily removed once placed and lasts up to 2 years. As such, it is recommended for the experienced patient in whom one is attempting to fill a deeper fold, with overlying thick skin. If Radiesse is placed superficially, the white paste-like substance can be seen through the translucent skin. This effect is true for superficially placed hyalurons as well, leading to a bluish coloration (Tyndall effect). However, in the case of the hyalurons, the filler can be dissolved readily if needed.

Voluma (Allergan) is the latest hyaluron to reach the US market. Allergan claims that this filler has a specific V-cross technology that provides for longer-lasting fill. It is approved by the Food and Drug Administration (FDA) for facial augmentation in the malar region.

Sculptra, or poly-L-lactic acid, is a particle injected in a highly diluted solution of saline and lidocaine to volumize the deflation that defines aging. The particle is mixed into a colloidal suspension (think shaken snow globe) and injected throughout the face, especially in areas of significant atrophy, such as the temples, malar eminence, and nasojugal folds. The diluent disappears within 24 hours, leaving the widely dispersed particles available for neocollagenesis. The effect from Sculptra takes several months to develop with the increase in newly synthesized collagen, and generally multiple injections are required, spaced out over 6 to 12 months for optimal results.

The following sections list fillers recommended according to type of rhytid needing correction.

Mild to Moderate Rhytids

Restylane was designed to be injected into the mid to deep dermal layers of the skin and was FDA approved in 2003 for treatment of mild to moderate wrinkle reduction. It received FDA approval in 2011 for lip augmentation. Restylane has a particle size of 300 microns. The hyaluronic acid (HA) concentration of Restylane is 20 mg/mL. Seventy-five percent of this exists in the cross-linked gel, while 25% is not cross-linked to decrease viscosity (15 mg/mL of HA). This product is designed to last between 9 to 12 months.

Juvéderm has a higher of concentration of HA than Restylane (24 mg/mL of HA). However, 60% of Juvéderm exists as a cross-linked gel (12 mg/mL of HA). The difference between Juvéderm Ultra and Juvéderm Ultra Plus is in the percentage of cross-linking between the HA molecules. Juvéderm has 2% cross-linking, Juvéderm Ultra has 6% cross-linking, and Juvéderm Ultra Plus has 8% cross-linking. Cross-linking increases the viscosity of the compound. An increase in viscosity promotes greater fill for deeper rhytids. Juvéderm Ultra XC and Juvéderm Ultra Plus XC contain 0.3% lidocaine in a physiologic buffer. The particle size of Juvéderm and Restylane is identical (300 microns).

Restylane-L and Juvéderm XC, both of which contain 0.3% lidocaine are my products of choice for mild to moderate rhytids and lip augmentation, especially for first-time users.

Moderate Rhytids

Perlane is about 3 times thicker than Restylane and is useful for deeper folds (nasolabial) and volume augmentation (lips). Perlane has an HA concentration of 20 mg/mL and larger particle size (650 micron). It is a good choice for deep nasolabial fold correction, and may be injected below the dermis in the preperiosteal plane to correct deeper volume deficits. As is true for Restylane and all the hyalurons, Perlane can be dissipated with an injection of hyaluronidase if the filler treatment requires adjustment.

Marketed for moderate to deep lines, Belotero Balance was FDA approved in 2011. Belotero Balance is a bacterial-derived hyaluron with an HA concentration of 22.5 mg/mL designed to integrate into the facial skin. Belotero Balance does not contain lidocaine, but may be used in combination with topical anesthetic products or region nerve blocks. The product is approved for moderate nasolabial folds but may be appropriate for delicate smile lines, vertical lip lines, or tear trough depressions.

Deep Rhytids

The heavier fillers are useful for the correction of moderate to deep facial rhytids. Radiesse, or calcium hydroxyapatite, was FDA approved for wrinkle reduction in 2006. Radiesse is composed of 25- to 45-micron microspheres of calcium hydroxyapatite suspended in a carboxymethylcellulose gel. The average longevity of fill is 12 to 18 months. Once injected, the carboxymethylcellulose gel dissolves, leaving the calcium hydroxyapatite to serve as a scaffold to promote fibroblast ingrowth and collagen formation.

Radiesse should be injected in the deep dermal or subdermal plane because more superficial injection may lead to white deposits visible beneath the surface of the skin. Given this risk, Radiesse should not be used for lip augmentation. Radiesse use should be limited to experienced injectors and patients. Unlike the hyalurons, there is no current method for removal of material once injected.

Global Volumization

Current aesthetic research describes the overall facial deflation that occurs with age. Rather than fill a single line or fold, specific fillers provide for overall facial volumization.

Sculptra, or poly-L-lactic acid (PLLA), is a suspension of particles injected globally to provide a dispersed scaffold for collagenesis. Sculptra was FDA approved for treatment of HIV-associated lipodystrophy in 2004 and for aesthetic use in 2009. The PLLA microspheres are 40 to 63 microns in size and are injected in the deep dermis or preperiosteal plane. Sculptra is a powder that must be diluted with saline and local anesthetic at least 24 hours prior to injection. Once injected, the diluent is absorbed within 24 hours; however, the enhanced collagen formation lasts about 24 months. Because of the risk for nodule formation, Sculptra should be maximally diluted and recipients instructed to massage their face 5 times a day, for 5 minutes, for 5 days to avoid nodule formation.

Juvéderm Voluma XC received FDA approval in October 2013. Juvéderm Voluma XC is a sterile, biodegradable, viscoelastic gel implant. It consists of Vycross-linked HA produced by *Streptococcus equii* bacteria, formulated to a concentration of 20 mg/mL with 0.3% lidocaine. Juvéderm Voluma XC is injected into facial tissue to temporarily restore volume and fullness to the areas of the midface. Voluma lasts up to 2 years. Patients may experience moderate tenderness, swelling, firmness, and/or lumps and bumps at the injection site, which generally last 2 to 4 weeks.

Artefill, which has changed its name to Bellafill, is a nonresorbable injectable dermal filler for the correction of wrinkles and lines on the face. Bellafill was approved by the FDA for correcting nasolabial folds but it is widely used off label. It is a formulation of medical grade polymethylmethacrylate (PMMA) microspheres and bovine collagen along with lidocaine and buffers. The PMMA microspheres in Bellafill are not absorbed by the body and therefore provide permanent support for wrinkle correction. Bellafill requires skin testing because its collagen base is of bovine origin. Given this, as well as the permanent nature of the PMMA microspheres, Bellafill is not my product of choice.

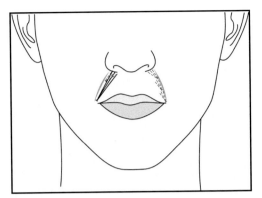

Figure 5-1. Serial puncture, threading technique for nasojugal folds.

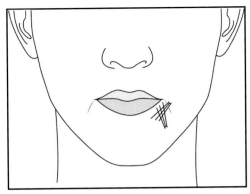

Figure 5-2. Cross-hatch technique for marionette lines.

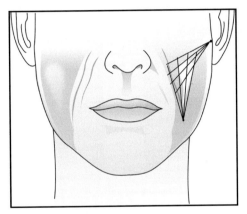

Figure 5-3. Midface augmentation technique.

Allopathic Fillers

The use of fat injection as well as autologous cultured human fibroblasts (LaViv) are techniques that attempt to replenish and restore fat, stem cells, or fibroblasts to aging skin.

Fat is considered a desirable filler—certainly most people are happy to be donors—and may be optimal for facial rejuvenation. However, periocular fat injections are very temperamental. The thin eyelid skin ensures that this technique is unforgiving. Additionally, as the fat is taken from the abdomen or buttock, both areas susceptible to fluctuation with weight gain, the injected facial fat may change in both size and configuration with weight variations. Removal of facial fat, especially around the eyes, is not easy.

Currently, all fillers have limitations, whether they be synthetic or autogenous. The skillful injector is able to approach the task of facial rejuvenation with an artistic eye and select the filler most suited to the needs of the individual. Depending on the facial contours and financial limitations of the patient, an individualized filler service can be developed. There are several techniques available for filler delivery such as serial point injection, threading, cross-hatching, and volumizing. Figures 5-1 through 5-3 demonstrate these techniques. Figure 5-4 shows pre- and postinjection examples of Restylane used to treat nasojugal folds, and Figure 5-5 shows pre- and postinjection examples of Sculptra for midface lipoatrophy.

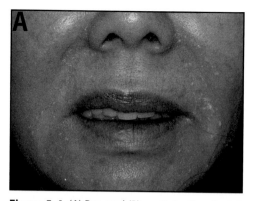 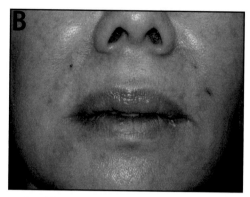

Figure 5-4. (A) Pre- and (B) postinjection Restylane for nasojugal line correction.

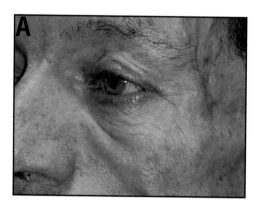 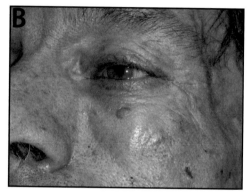

Figure 5-5. (A) Pre- and (B) postinjection of Sculptra for midface augmentation.

It is recommended that the injector become familiar with a limited cohort of products initially, each specific for a superficial or deep rhytid, as well as overall volumization. Once the use of a select group of fillers has been mastered, additional fillers can be added to the injector's armamentarium of aesthetic rejuvenative tools.

Bibliography

Allemann I, Baumann L. Hyaluronic acid gel (Juvéderm) preparations in the treatment of facial wrinkles and folds. *Clin Interv Aging.* 2008;3(4):629-634.

Funt D, Pavicic T. Dermal filler in aesthetics: an overview of adverse events and treatment approaches. *Clin Cosmet Investig Dermatol.* 2013;(6):295-316.

Kablik J, Monheit GD, Yu L, Chang G, Gershkovich J. Comparative physical properties of hyaluronic acid dermal fillers. *Dermatol Surg.* 2009;(35):302-312.

Lipham W, Melicher J. *Clinical Applications of Botox and Dermal Fillers.* 3rd ed. Thorofare, NJ: SLACK Incorporated; 2015.

WHAT LASERS ARE AVAILABLE AND WHICH DO YOU PREFER FOR FACIAL RESURFACING?

Wendy W. Lee, MD, MS; Audrey C. Ko, MD; and Marcus J. Ko, MD

How are lasers used in oculoplastic surgery? Which patients are most likely to benefit from laser resurfacing? Do you have any suggestions to avoid complications?

Lasers are a versatile tool that can be used alone or in combination with topical treatments, injectables, and/or surgery for effective rejuvenation of the skin. Facial resurfacing by lasers is commonly used to address photoaging by improving the appearance of rhytids, pigmentary irregularities, acne or surgical scars, and skin tone. The two categories of lasers used in facial resurfacing are ablative and nonablative lasers. Current devices include, but are not limited to, those listed in Table 6-1. Selection of the type of laser and treatment regimen needs to be customized to each patient because each type of laser has distinct advantages and disadvantages.

Starting with the least invasive, the 1064-nm nonfractional, nonablative laser platform (Laser Genesis, Cutera) is at the most conservative end of the spectrum. No pretreatment topical anesthetic is required and posttreatment side effects are minimal, which is why it is sometimes called a lunchtime procedure. Patients have minimal discomfort during treatment because the handpiece does not come into contact with the skin, but rather is waved 1 to 2 cm above the skin like a wand to deliver heat. The laser is delivered in micropulse duration to heat the treated dermis, resulting in dermal collagen production and the reduction of fine wrinkles and improved skin tone. The downside of this gentler modality is it requires a greater number of treatments to achieve results (at least 6), but the advantage is it can be used in any skin type.

The next step up is nonablative fractional laser (NAFL), such as the 1550-nm laser (Fraxel) and other similar platforms. NAFL delivers laser energy to the dermis in noncontiguous columns of microthermal treatment zones (MTZ) of injury with intervening untreated dermis.[1] This results in what is called fractional thermolysis, which stimulates collagen production and reduces dyspigmentation. Not only is this laser effective on the face, but it can also be used on the neck, chest,

Kersten RC, McCulley TJ, eds. *Curbside Consultation in Oculoplastics:*
49 Clinical Questions, Second Edition (pp 33-37).
© 2016 Taylor & Francis Group.

Table 6-1
Examples of Ablative and Nonablative Lasers Used in Facial Resurfacing[3]

Ablative Lasers			
Wavelength	**Laser Type**	**Company**	**Device Name**
2790 nm	Erbium:YSGG	Cutera	Pearl
2790 nm	Erbium:YSGG (fractional)	Cutera	Pearl Fractional
2940 nm	Erbium:YAG	Sciton	Contour TRL
2940 nm	Erbium:YAG (fractional)	Sciton	Profractional
2940 nm	Erbium:YAG (fractional)	Palomar	Lux2940
10,600 nm	CO_2	Lumenis	Active FX
10,600 nm	CO_2 (fractional)	Lumenis	Deep FX
10,600 nm	CO_2 (fractional)	Solta	Fraxel re:pair
Nonablative Lasers			
Wavelength	**Laser Type**	**Company**	**Device Name**
1064 nm	YAG	Cutera	Laser Genesis
1410 nm	Diode (fractional)	Palomar	Emerge
1440 nm	Diode (fractional)	Solta	Clear and Brilliant
1540 nm	Erbium (fractional)	Palomar	Lux1540
1550 nm	Erbium Glass Fiber (fractional)	Solta	Fraxel re:store

YSGG = Yttrium-scandium-gallium-garnet; YAG = Yttrium-aluminum-garnet; CO_2 = carbon dioxide.

hands, and eyelids, among other areas. When used on the eyelids, patients notice a tightening of the skin and reduction in dark circles. This laser is a good choice for patients with skin types I to IV (Table 6-2) and those who would like more aggressive treatment with more significant results than nonfractional nonablative laser, but without the downtime required with ablative laser resurfacing. Like the Laser Genesis, nonablative fractional lasers also require a series of treatments for optimal results (on average 3 to 6). Posttreatment, patients may be red and swollen for a few days, but this can be covered up with makeup because the stratum corneum remains intact. Posttreatment side effects are minimal. An example of pretreatment appearance and posttreatment results with reduction in fine lines and improved skin tone is shown in Figure 6-1.

The most aggressive laser treatments for skin resurfacing are the ablative lasers, which include wavelengths of 2790, 2940, and 10,600 nm (see Table 6-1). These lasers have a high affinity for water and cause vaporization and surrounding thermal necrosis when the energy is absorbed by the targeted tissue. Ablative lasers can also be used in 2 different ways: nonfractional and fractional. Nonfractional ablative treatment causes a superficial confluent laser injury to the epidermis and superficial dermis. In contrast, fractional treatment is delivered in nonconfluent, deeper, thinner

Table 6-2
Fitzpatrick Sun Reactive Skin Types[3]

Skin Phototypes	
Type I	
Pale white	Always burns, never tans
Type II	
White	Usually burns, tans minimally
Type III	
Light brown	Sometimes burns, tans uniformly
Type IV	
Moderate brown	Rarely burns, tans well
Type V	
Dark brown	Very rarely burns, tans easily
Type VI	
Black	Never burns, always tans

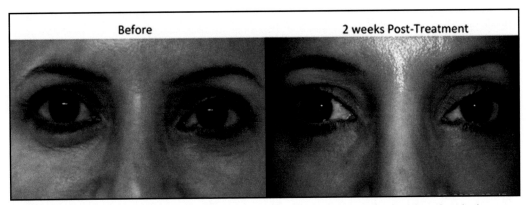

Figure 6-1. Before treatment with a nonablative fractional laser, the patient had fine rhytids that were most noticeable in the lower eyelid region. There was marked improvement in skin tone and appearance of fine rhytids after treatment.

columns with intervening normal, untreated skin. The normal untreated surrounding skin acts as a reservoir for healing, and promotes more rapid reepithelialization and recovery. The ablative lasers typically used in facial resurfacing include carbon dioxide and Erbium (eg, Er:YAG or Er:YSGG) lasers. Erbium lasers can be used to treat superficial and deep rhytids. CO_2 laser resurfacing is commonly used to treat deep rhytids, scars, and enlarged pores. Compared to the CO_2 laser, the erbium laser has a higher affinity for water and therefore has less bulk heating and fewer potential risks. Ablative lasers are safest when used in skin types I to III (see Table 6-2). They may not require as many treatments as the nonablative lasers (usually 1 to 2 depending on

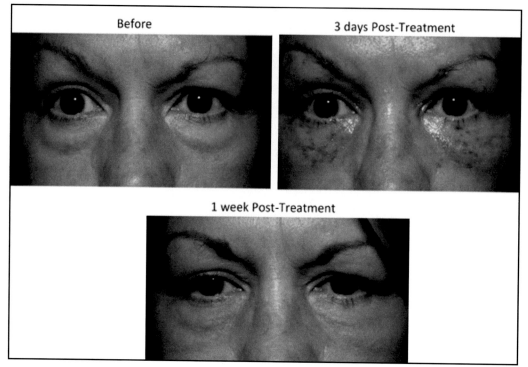

Figure 6-2. Before treatment with an ablative laser, the patient had fine rhytids and loose skin tone. In the lower eyelid region, the loose skin tone and prolapse of orbital fat resulted in the appearance of undereye circles. Three days after treatment with an ablative laser, the patient had erythema in the treated areas, which is expected after this procedure. It was markedly improved by postoperative week 1. At 1 week after treatment, there is a large improvement in skin tone and appearance of rhytids despite posttreatment edema.

the aggressiveness of the settings), but the downtime is longer. Ablative lasers can also be used on the face and on the eyelids for tightening, thickening of the skin, and decrease in fine wrinkles.[4] An example of pretreatment appearance, immediate posttreatment appearance, and posttreatment results with reduction of the appearance of rhytids and improved skin tone using fractional ablative laser resurfacing is shown in Figure 6-2.

Prior to laser resurfacing, there are several important factors to consider in the evaluation of patients. Darker skin types have a higher risk of postinflammatory hyperpigmentation (PIH). This risk can be minimized by using nonablative treatments or by pre- and posttreating with a tyrosinase inhibitor, such as hydroquinone. Patients with a history of inflammatory (eg, eczema and psoriasis), autoimmune (eg, lupus), or infectious skin disorders (eg, herpes simplex virus, molluscum) may experience worsening of their condition after treatment.[2] There is some belief that photosensitizing medications (eg, topical tretinoin) and blood thinning medications (eg, aspirin, ibuprofen, and vitamin E) should be stopped prior to treatment, but our experience does not strongly endorse this practice. Risks such as burns, scarring, hyper- or hypopigmentation, and infection should be discussed with the patient. It is also recommended that patients with a history of herpes simplex virus are treated with prophylactic oral antiviral agents prior to ablative laser treatment, and that patients with active infections are treated prior to ablative facial resurfacing.[2]

Patients undergoing both nonablative (with the exception of Laser Genesis) and ablative laser treatments need application of a topical anesthetic cream (eg, topical lidocaine 5% cream) for 45 to 60 minutes prior to treatment. Sedation can be used with CO_2 or erbium treatments, but are also tolerable in many patients without. Application of cool air during and after the treatment assists in reducing patient discomfort. A smoke evacuator must be used with the ablative lasers to absorb the plume that is created.

Settings can be chosen depending on the targeted pathology and vary from platform to platform. The parameters that are most commonly adjusted are energy and density. The energy corresponds to the depth of treatment and the density or level corresponds to the percentage of treated skin per treatment spot. Energy should be increased when treating deeper wrinkles or acne scars, whereas energy can be decreased for superficial conditions, such as melasma. Density should be chosen based on the desired aggressiveness of the treatment. A higher density positively correlates with more effective results, but has more associated patient discomfort and risk, such as postinflammatory hyperpigmentation. One approach is to start with a conservative density and increase based on the patient's response to the first treatment. Spot size can also be varied on each unit to fit the area to be treated.

Before treatment, it is important to warn your patient of what to expect. Lasers, especially ablative, can be loud and potentially startling, and some prefer to wear earplugs. During laser treatment, the patient may experience a pinprick sensation even after application of topical anesthetic. Knowing this ahead of time will set the patient's expectations and may reduce anxiety during the treatment.

Patients should receive appropriate posttreatment counseling as well. With ablative lasers, they should expect mild pain, swelling, pinpoint bleeding, or serous oozing from the treated areas immediately following treatment and during the recovery period. Bland ointment (eg, Aquaphor ointment or Vaseline) is applied to the treated area 3 times a day until epithelialization. It is not necessary to apply topical antibiotics. In fact, any topicals prior to reepithelialization must be used with caution given the high risk for a contact dermatitis after ablative lasers. After reepithelialization, which takes usually 4 to 7 days, topical creams, cleansers, and makeup can be resumed. The use of a broad-spectrum sunscreen that blocks ultraviolet A and B rays is recommended as well. Nonablative lasers, as mentioned above, generally only cause mild redness and swelling for a few days. Topicals and makeup can be applied immediately after treatment. Repeat treatments can be performed as early as 1 month. Once desired results are achieved, many patients may wish to have yearly maintenance treatments.

Laser skin resurfacing is an effective tool to rejuvenate the face and has become increasingly popular amongst the nonsurgical aesthetic procedures around the world. It is best used in combination with other aesthetic treatments such as injectables (eg, botulinum toxins or fillers) and surgery because each addresses a different aspect of rejuvenation, with lasers having the greatest ability to address the quality of the skin. There are many modalities and units available that will provide visible results. Becoming familiar with the technology and incorporating lasers into an aesthetic practice provides patients with a comprehensive menu of available aesthetic procedures that can lead to an optimal outcome.

References

1. Thomas JR, Somenek M. Journal club: scar revision review. *Arch Facial Plast Surg.* 2012;14(3):162-174.
2. Metelitsa AI, Alster TS. Fractionated laser skin resurfacing treatment complications: a review. *Dermatol Surg.* 2010;36(3):299-306.
3. Fitzpatrick TB. The validity and practicality of sun-reactive skin types I through VI. *Arch Dermatol.* 1988;124(6):869-871.
4. Goldman MP, Fitzpatrick RE, Ross EV, Kilmer SL, Weiss RA, eds. *Lasers and Energy Devices for the Skin.* 2nd ed. Boca Raton: CRC Press; 2013.

WHAT IS THE DIFFERENCE BETWEEN LASER RESURFACING AND CHEMICAL PEELS?

Jerry K. Popham, MD, FACS

What are the indications for these techniques? Which do you prefer? Do you ever perform resurfacing at the same time as a blepharoplasty? Is there anything wrong with staging blepharoplasty and resurfacing?

Although skin rejuvenation techniques probably began centuries ago in ancient Egypt, recent advances have given physicians many options for improving the quality of their patients' skin. Skin resurfacing is directed toward the removal of the surface skin, resulting in the growth of new, fresher skin whose appearance is rejuvenated. These techniques are used to remove superficial dyschromias and textural abnormalities, as well as deeper rhytids and scars. Successful rejuvenation requires that this be accomplished without visible scarring or hyper- or hypopigmentation. In addition, more invasive skin ablation requires deeper anesthesia and risks reactivation of herpetic skin infection or de novo bacterial infection. For these reasons, recent resurfacing techniques have trended toward less ablative methodologies. Skin resurfacing and rejuvenation techniques may be classified into 3 major categories: mechanical, chemical, and laser.

Mechanical Techniques

Mechanical techniques include dermaplaning, dermabrasion, microdermabrasion, and microneedle roller devices. Dermaplaning involves the superficial removal of epithelium using a surgical scalpel and a planing technique. Dermabrasion techniques are relatively aggressive and are typically performed in the operating room under general or monitored anesthesia care. Dermabrasion is directed toward deep scarring such as traumatic scars or the scarring resulting from high-grade cystic acne. Fortunately, this type of scarring is becoming less common due to such acne preventive treatments as isotretinoin. Dermabrasion uses wire brushes or abrasive

Kersten RC, McCulley TJ, eds. *Curbside Consultation in Oculoplastics:*
49 Clinical Questions, Second Edition (pp 39-41).
© 2016 Taylor & Francis Group.

surfaces to sand away the epidermis and superficial dermis, inducing reformation of new superficial dermis and epidermis with a smoother surface. Microdermabrasion techniques are significantly less aggressive than dermabrasion techniques and use an abrasive substance such as silica crystals to resurface the skin by mechanically removing the surface cells. The microdermabrasion techniques generally penetrate to a minimal depth and therefore have less benefit than other techniques. Microneedle rollers are devices involving hundreds of very fine needles of varying lengths on a cylindrical roller. The needles are rolled over the skin and penetrate to the depth of the needle. These devices have been shown to be effective in reducing scarring, pigmentary changes, and fine rhytids. The microneedle rollers may be combined with the use of various topical medications, whose penetrance is greatly enhanced after the skin is penetrated by the needles.

Chemical Techniques

Chemical techniques are categorized based on the depth of peeling (ie, superficial, intermediate, and deep). Deeper peels result in more impressive improvement in wrinkles, but also result in more prolonged erythema, delayed healing, and carry a greater risk for hyper- or hypopigmentation and scarring. In experienced and knowledgeable hands, it is usually possible to induce skin sloughing and rejuvenation to the desired depth without significant thermal injury, hypopigmentation, or scarring. Static wrinkles are generally targeted through the use of chemical peels, whereas dynamic wrinkles are typically best addressed through the use of neurotoxins.

Penetrance from superficial peels is minimal, and these peels act essentially as exfoliants. Examples include the lunchtime peel that is typically an alpha hydroxyl acid or glycolic acid peel. Superficial peels, by definition, penetrate only to the epidermis. Medium depth peels, such as trichloroacetic acid (TCA) peels and the TCA variant, Obagi Blue Peel, penetrate the epidermis to the superficial dermis and papillary dermis and are generally directed toward reducing fine lines and superficial pigment changes. Deep chemical peels, typically using phenol with croton oil, penetrate to the reticular dermis and, depending on the aggressiveness of the peel, may be quite effective in reducing fine and medium depth rhytids and deeper pigmentary changes.

Manual application of chemical peels can be somewhat imprecise with variable concentration and distribution of chemical across the surface to be treated, so a more uniform ablation by laser resurfacing is often preferred. Pigmentary disturbances after chemical or laser resurfacing are more pronounced in darker pigmented skin, and may include hyper- or hypopigmentation. For this reason, treatment with most resurfacing methods is restricted to use in Fitzpatrick type I to IV skin. Fortunately, photoaging is less pronounced in patients with Fitzpatrick type V to VI skin.

Laser Techniques

Laser skin rejuvenation techniques have advanced dramatically in the past decade and are further covered in Chapter 6. Carbon dioxide laser resurfacing was introduced in the mid-1990s. The CO_2 laser has a wavelength of 10,660 nm, which is absorbed by water, resulting in vaporization of the surface soft tissue. This causes an aggressive sloughing of the treated surface and initially its use in a continuous treatment mode resulted in prolonged erythema, frequent permanent hypopigmentation, and occasional scarring. For this reason, a number of alternative laser modalities have been developed. Generally, these modalities have been directed toward using lasers with different wavelengths (erbium or yttrium, scandium, gallium, garnet laser), and varying energy intensity, duration (pulsing), or surface exposure (fractionating). The goal of these variations has been to attempt to achieve similar rejuvenation, while reducing the risks and longer recovery time associated with the more invasive continuous CO_2 laser exposure. Laser resurfacing offers the advantage of very accurate depths of penetrance based on the settings programmed into the machine and the wavelength of the specific laser. More sophisticated pattern generators allow more even application of laser energy, thus reducing excessive thermal energy exposure with resultant scarring. The CO_2 laser has been modified by delivering short pulses of laser energy that vaporize tissue without causing as much thermal damage. A more recent innovation is the fractionating of surface treatments so that a pattern generator results in treatment of only 5% to 30% of the total surface area of the skin at one sitting. This can still be programmed to penetrate to variable depths based on the patient's skin type, skin problems, and goals. Fractional treatment results in ablation of columns of dermis/epidermis without harming the surrounding skin. Because only a small percentage of the skin surface is ablated, the skin reepithelializes rapidly, offering faster recovery times. Fractionated laser treatments can usually be administered with just topical anesthesia, obviating the need for general or monitored sedation. On the other hand, multiple treatments are required to achieve significant improvement.

Summary

Chemical peeling and laser resurfacing are indicated for patients with static facial rhytids, superficial dyschromias, textural abnormalities, and scars. Chemical peeling techniques may be applied to virtually all body surfaces with proper dosage and application technique, but laser resurfacing is primarily directed to facial skin. Resurfacing with either chemical or laser technique is commonly combined with blepharoplasty or with face and neck lifting, with certain limitations. Surgical excision of skin and lifting of facial or eyelid structures implies skin tightening, which is also an effect of laser or chemical peeling. To avoid excessive skin tightening or even cicatricial ectropion, the surgeon must judge the combined effects of the surgical, chemical, and laser techniques to avoid the complications of overtightening. Some surgeons stage skin resurfacing and surgery by using skin resurfacing techniques a few weeks prior to the surgical procedure, thus reducing the chance of overcorrection.

Suggested Readings

Deprez P. *Textbook of Chemical Peels. Superficial, Medium, and Deep Peels in Cosmetic Practice*. UK: Informa Healthcare; 2007.

Fischer TC, Perosino E, Poli F, Viera MS, Dreno B, Cosmetic Dermatology European Expert Group. Chemical peels in aesthetic dermatology: an update 2009. *J Eur Acad Dermatol Venereol*. 2010;24(3):281-292.

Holck DE, Ng JD. Facial skin rejuvenation. *Curr Opin Ophthalmol*. 2003;14:246-252.

Rohrich RJ, Herbig KS. The role of modified Jessner's solution with 35% trichloroacetic acid peel. *Plast Reconstr Surg*. 2009;124(3):965-966.

WHAT ALTERNATIVES TO BOTOX ARE AVAILABLE AND HOW DO THEY COMPARE?

Timothy J. McCulley, MD; W. Jordan Piluek, MD;
and Lynda V. McCulley, PharmD

I've been hearing about alternatives to Botox. Can you tell me what the difference is? Which do you prefer?

The bacteria *Clostridium botulinum* produces numerous toxins. Botulinum toxin type A (BTA) is 1 of 8. It acts by inhibiting the release of acetylcholine (ACh).[1] As you may recall from your medical school neurology class, striated muscles and the targets of the parasympathetic nervous system use cholinergic receptors. Postganglionic sympathetic neurons are adrenergic, with the exception of sweat glands, which are cholinergic. Therefore, BTA effectively inhibits striated muscles (eg, orbicularis oculi, brow depressors, extraocular muscles), parasympathetically inner-vated glands (eg, the lacrimal gland), and sweat glands (ie, treatment of axillary hyperhidrosis).

BTA is most commonly marketed under the trade name Botox (the registered trade name of Allergan, Inc). The number of competing commercial BTA products available is rapidly increasing, each with elaborate marketing campaigns. Not only are the number of companies that produce BTA multiplying, the same drug may go by more than one name. For example, BTXA is produced by a Chinese company. Alternate brand names for the same medication include Prosigne when sold in Brazil, Redux when sold in Peru, Lantox when sold in Russia and Colombia, and Lanzox in Indonesia. Keeping them straight and sorting through the advertising nonsense is becoming more of a challenge.

A distinguishing characteristic is potency of a unit of drug. BTA is calibrated in somewhat arbitrary units. One unit corresponds to the median lethal intraperitoneal dose (LD50) in mice. Although the mouse LD50 is used as the measure of a unit in both Botox and Dysport, the poten-cies of these 2 products differ. Although debated, in humans 1 unit of Botox is probably about 2.5 times more potent than a single unit of Dysport. This difference is a result of each company having its own nuances of testing the ill-fated mice. Some might prefer one product to the other, but when dose adjusted, you can probably expect similar results between products. Most other BTA brands have dosing comparable with that of Botox (Table 8-1).

Kersten RC, McCulley TJ, eds. *Curbside Consultation in Oculoplastics:*
49 Clinical Questions, Second Edition (pp 43-45).
© 2016 Taylor & Francis Group.

Table 8-1
Commercially Available Botulinum Toxins

Trade Name(s)	Manufacturer	Approved in the USA	Active Ingredient	Dose*	Mean Duration
Botox	Allergan	Yes	Botulinum toxin A	1 unit	3 months
Xeomin+	Merz	Yes	Botulinum toxin A	1 unit	3 months
Dysport	Medicis	Yes	Botulinum toxin A	2 to 3 units	3 to 4 months
Purtox++	Mentor	No	Botulinum toxin A	1 unit	3 months
BTXA (Lantox, Prosigne)+++	LIBP	No	Botulinum toxin A	1 unit	3 months
Neuronox (Siax)	Medy-Tox	No	Botulinum toxin A	1 unit	3 months
Myobloc (Neurobloc)	Solstice Neurosciences	Yes	Botulinum toxin B	16 units	Less than 3 months

* = number of units equivalent to 1unit of Botox; + Xeomin claims to use a unique proprietary purification process to remove accessory proteins from botulinum toxin type A; ++ Purtox, even prior to FDA approval, has been marketed as another pure form of BTA, with the alleged benefit of being quicker acting and longer lasting, an unsubstantiated claim common amongst Botox competitors;
+++ = BTXA claims to use bovine gelatin as a substitute for albumin, commonly used in other formulations; LIBP = Lanzhou Institute of Biological Products

The most common marketing ploy is to claim varying degrees of purity. The idea is that by purifying the BTA, one reduces the immune reaction to the drug. This is then claimed to have a number of benefits such as quicker action, longer duration, and less likelihood of developing resistance. There are little to no bias-free data available to substantiate these claims and it is our impression that whatever benefits purification offers will likely prove negligible.

In our opinion, the most substantial differences between brands of BTA are pricing and the quantity that is available for purchase. Previously, Botox was only available in 100-unit vials and recommended for single use, so if a patient only needed a small amount, there were large amounts of waste. Today, companies offer a wide variety of quantities. This is changing so frequently that we are hesitant to catalog what is available currently. Our suggestion is to check with your institution or local pharmacy and go with whatever quantity is most economical.

Myobloc (Solstice Neurosciences, Inc) is a slightly different drug. It is botulinum toxin type B (BTB). Myobloc is a unique product in that its active ingredient is BTB as opposed to all the others, which are type A. The mechanism of BTB is similar to that of BTA, with the exception that BTB cleaves the protein VAMP, whereas BTA cleaves SNAP-25. Our impression of Myobloc is that the injections are more painful. A much larger dose in terms of units is needed, making dose adjustment difficult for those of us used to using Botox. Our impression is also that it does not seem to work quite as well and does not last as long. The benefit of Myobloc is that it may remain effective in patients who have developed immune mediated resistance to BTA. We have never used Myobloc for cosmetic purposes and reserve its use for patients with blepharospasm (or related diseases) in whom BTA has become ineffective.

Summary

BTA earns its popularity. It is our preferred treatment modality for blepharospasm and related disorders and can be an attractive cosmetic adjunct.[2-4] The market is currently being flooded with products and clever advertisements. Dysport is unique in that the potency of 1 unit is less than that of other products. Myobloc is truly unique in that it is comprised of BTB and, in our practice, serves only as backup to BTA should resistance develop. Our impression is that the efficacies of most BTA products are indistinguishable. Until proven otherwise, our advice is to select the product that offers the best value.

References

1. Scott AB. Development of botulinum toxin therapy. *Dermatol Clin.* 2004;22(2):131-133.
2. Dutton JJ, Fowler AM. Botulinum toxin in ophthalmology. *Focal points: Clinical Modules for Ophthalmologists.* San Francisco: American Academy of Ophthalmology; 2007.
3. McCulley TJ, Hwang TN. Blepharospasm. In Lee AG, Brazis PW, Kline LB, eds. *Curbside Consultation in Neuro-ophthalmology: 49 Clinical Questions.* Thorofare, NJ: SLACK Incorporated; 2008.
4. McCulley TJ, Yoon MK. How do you use Botox? In Kersten RC, McCulley TJ, eds. *Curbside Consultation in Oculoplastics: 49 Clinical Questions.* Thorofare, NJ: SLACK Incorporated; 2010.

SECTION II

EYELID

WHEN SHOULD I BE CONCERNED ABOUT SYSTEMIC DISEASE IN A PATIENT WITH BLEPHAROPTOSIS?

Robert C. Kersten, MD, FACS and
Chris Thiagarajah, MD, FACS

I'm worried that my patient with blepharoptosis has myasthenia gravis. When is additional evaluation warranted and what test(s) should I order? What other conditions might be missed in a patient with blepharoptosis?

Most often, acquired blepharoptosis is due to involutional changes of the levator muscle or its aponeurosis.[1] However, many other etiologies need to be considered. Numerous serious neurological and systemic diseases can result in blepharoptosis.[2] Table 9-1 lists some of the diseases to be considered. Most can be identified with a thorough evaluation.

Always start with a thorough history. A history of intraocular surgery, previous trauma, or rigid contact lens wear suggests levator dehiscence. When did the ptosis occur? Blepharoptosis with an acute or subacute onset suggests a neurological problem such as Horner syndrome, a third nerve palsy, or myasthenia gravis. Gradual onset is more consistent with involutional or age-related blepharoptosis.

All patients with blepharoptosis should be asked about diplopia. Diplopia is common, but not necessarily present in all patients with myasthenia gravis. It is present in binocular patients with oculomotor nerve paresis unless the eyelid completely occludes the visual axis or the patient did not have single binocular vision prior to its onset. Variability of the blepharoptosis is the hallmark of myasthenia gravis. In these patients, other possible symptoms include improvement with rest, symptoms worse at the end of the day, and fatigue in other parts of the body. However, patients who have involutional blepharoptosis may also complain of fatigability. This is because these patients usually recruit the ipsilateral frontalis muscle to compensate for the lower eyelid height and this can lead to fatigue at the end of the day. Many of these patients also complain of worsening of ptosis when reading because it is difficult to elevate the brow in downgaze.

Kersten RC, McCulley TJ, eds. *Curbside Consultation in Oculoplastics:*
49 Clinical Questions, Second Edition (pp 49-54).
© 2016 Taylor & Francis Group.

Table 9-1
Neuromuscular Diseases Associated With Blepharoptosis

Myogenic
- Congential
- Muscular dystrophy
- Chronic progressive external ophthalmoplegia
- Congenital fibrosis of the extraocular muscles

Oculomotor Nerve
- Compressive
- Ischemic
- Traumatic

Neuromuscular Junction
- Myasthenia gravis
- Lambert-Eaton syndrome

Sympathetic Nervous System
- Horner syndrome

Synkinesis
- Facial nerve palsy
- Marcus Gunn jaw-winking syndrome
- Duane syndrome

Diffuse Neuromuscular Disease
- Amyotrophic lateral sclerosis

A complete ophthalmic examination should be performed on all patients, with particular attention to the pupil and motility evaluation. Horner's patients are expected to have anisocoria with a small pupil on the affected side. This anisocoria is expected to be worse in the dark. A larger pupil on the affected side suggests oculomotor nerve dysfunction. When accompanied by characteristic motility abnormalities, consideration should be given to computed tomography-angiography to evaluate for a posterior communicating artery aneurysm in the circle of Willis. Abnormalities in extraocular motility are not a surprise in patients with a third nerve palsy or myasthenia. Commonly, in myasthenics, there can be variability in the eye motility exam, and eye alignment measurements can be seen to vary even during the course of one exam. In any patient with associated abnormalities in extraocular motility, other cranial nerves should also be evaluated. A slit lamp exam may reveal other causes of blepharoptosis, such as superior limbic keratoconjunctivitis or follicles from ocular allergy or soft contact lens wear. Evaluate the undersurface of the eyelids for tarsal conjunctiva follicles or a displaced contact lens (Figure 9-1).

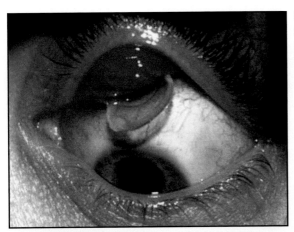

Figure 9-1. Unilateral acquired blepharoptosis. Giant papillary conjunctivitis in a young patient with a displaced contact lens that had been "lost" several weeks prior.

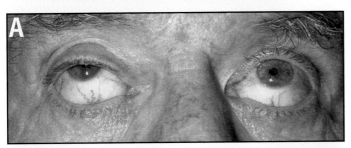

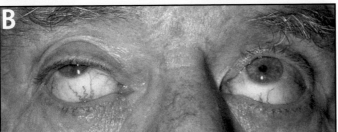

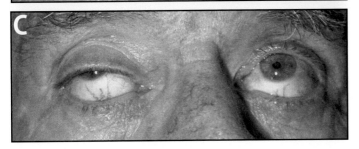

Figure 9-2. Fatigue test for myasthenia gravis. (A) A patient with acquired unilateral blepharoptosis in upgaze. (B) As the eyelid fatigues, the ptosis worsens 30 seconds later and (C) 60 seconds later.

In our experience, myasthenia gravis is the most commonly overlooked disease in patients referred with blepharoptosis. We recommend performing a fatigue test in all patients. This involves having the patient sustain upgaze for 30 seconds. As patients with ocular myasthenia fatigue, their ptosis should worsen (Figure 9-2). Alternatively, a rest test can be done by having the patient close both eyes for 15 minutes and reexamining the ptosis to see if it improves. Placing a bag of ice over the affected eyelid for 2 minutes will usually improve myasthenic ptosis (Figure 9-3).[3] Patients may also present with orbicularis weakness or a positive Cogan lid twitch sign. If

Figure 9-3. Ice test for myasthenia gravis. Unilateral blepharoptosis secondary to myasthenia gravis (A) before and (B) after an ice test.

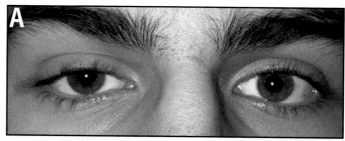
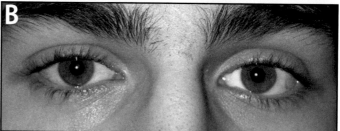

Figure 9-4. Cocaine testing for Horner syndrome. A young male with acquired unilateral blepharoptosis (A) before and (B) after placement of cocaine 10% drops.

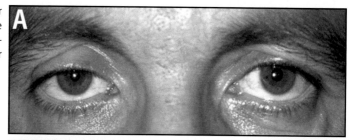
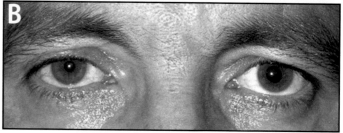

myasthenia is suspected, titers for acetylcholine receptor antibodies can be obtained. Keep in mind that they are positive in only half of patients with ocular myasthenia. For this reason, Tensilon testing remains the gold standard in the diagnosis. Another fairly sensitive test is single-fiber electromyography (EMG). If you suspect myasthenia gravis, we would recommend that you refer the patient to a neurologist who can help in selecting the appropriate test.

A mild blepharoptosis of up to 3 mm is seen in most cases of Horner syndrome. As mentioned, patients usually have miosis. Additionally, the patient may have elevation of the lower eyelid, often referred to as upside down ptosis. Depending on the level of the lesion, anhidrosis of the affected side of the face may be reported. Check intraocular pressure carefully. Mild relative hypotony of 1 to 3 mm Hg is usually seen on the affected side and may be a very helpful clue in more subtle cases. Cocaine testing is used to confirm the diagnosis of Horner syndrome (Figure 9-4). If cocaine is unavailable, recent investigations have found apraclonidine to be helpful in confirming the presence of Horner syndrome.[4] Apraclonidine, an α-adrenergic receptor agonist, has been reported to result in dilation of the miotic pupil due to denervation supersensitivity. However,

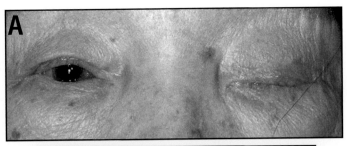

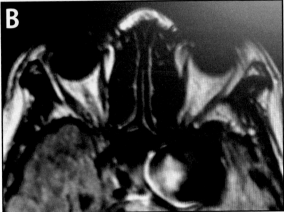

Figure 9-5. Compressive third nerve palsy. (A) An elderly female presented with severe acquired unilateral blepharoptosis secondary to a compressive third nerve palsy. Due to occlusion of the visual axis, she did not complain of diplopia; however, characteristic abnormal motility was easily identified with the extraocular motility evaluation. (B) Magnetic resonance imaging demonstrating a large thrombosed cavernous sinus aneurysm.

the true sensitivity of this test has been debated and its reliability remains to be confirmed. Hydroxyamphetamine can be used to distinguish third-order neuron abnormalities from first- and second-order neuron lesions. Magnetic resonance imaging from the hypothalamus to the lung apex, with angiography to assess for carotid artery dissection, will detect the vast majority of identifiable lesions.

A third nerve palsy is usually obvious due to the characteristic abnormalities in extraocular motility. Occasionally, in a monocular patient who does not report diplopia, a third nerve palsy might be missed. Also, patients with an eyelid so ptotic that the vision is occluded may not report diplopia (Figure 9-5). Traumatic and ischemic third nerve palsies are usually complete or near complete and not likely to be missed. However, compressive third nerve palsies are often initially only "partial" and may be overlooked. There have been a small handful of patients reported with blepharoptosis as an isolated finding due to a compressive lesion. This might be considered in a patient with no other explanation for unilateral blepharoptosis.

Summary

Although in most cases blepharoptosis is relatively benign, neuromuscular disease will occasionally be encountered. Be particularly suspicious in younger patients, those with unilateral ptosis, or with systemic symptoms or disease. Pay particular attention to the pupil and extraocular motility examinations. In all patients, inquire about symptoms of myasthenia gravis and test for fatigue and a Cogan lid twitch. Have a low threshold for additional testing.

References

1. Pereira LS, Hwang TN, Kersten RC, Ray K, McCulley TJ. Levator superioris muscle function in involutional blepharoptosis. *Am J Ophthalmol.* 2008;145:1095-1098.
2. Kersten RC, de Conciliis C, Kulwin DR. Acquired ptosis in the young and middle-aged adult populations. *Ophthalmology.* 1995;102:924-928.
3. Golnik KC, Pena R, Lee AG, Eggenberger ER. An ice test for the diagnosis of myasthenia gravis. *Ophthalmology.* 1999;106:1282-1286.
4. Antonio-Santos AA, Santo RN, Eggenberger ER. Pharmacological testing of anisocoria. *Expert Opin Pharmacother.* 2005;6:2007-2013.

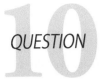
IS THERE EVER A GENETIC BASIS FOR ACQUIRED BLEPHAROPTOSIS?

Prem Subramanian, MD, PhD

The other day I saw and mother and her three adult children all with blepharoptosis, which began when each was a young adult. Could this be hereditary? Is there anything I should be concerned about?

When confronted with the patient who has acquired upper eyelid ptosis, the ophthalmologist routinely assesses several aspects of ocular and orbital health to arrive at the appropriate diagnosis. The following questions should be asked of the patient or considered during the initial evaluation:

- Is the ptosis unilateral or bilateral, and if bilateral is it symmetric?
- Is levator excursion normal, excessive (supranormal), or reduced?
- Are the pupils symmetric with equal reactivity and redilation?
- Are the eye movements and extraocular muscle balance normal?
- Is there a facial sensory deficit?
- Is there pseudoptosis because of contralateral eyelid retraction or ipsilateral enophthalmos?
- Does the ptosis vary diurnally?

Acquired ptosis from a genetic disorder may occur in isolation, but is more typically found with disorders of eye movement as well as other neuromuscular disturbances. Features of acquired ptosis that will increase suspicion for a genetic component include insidious onset (years) in a relatively asymptomatic patient; many individuals will develop a compensation strategy with a chin-up posture. In fact, some patients may have their ptosis diagnosed when they seek attention for their chronic neck pain. In other cases, patients present for ptosis evaluation because the eyelid change is noticed by friends or family, not by patients themselves. In addition, because the underlying conditions may be inherited in a mitochondrial or autosomal dominant fashion, the ptotic appearance may be considered a familial characteristic and not a disease state. It is quite unusual for ptosis to

Kersten RC, McCulley TJ, eds. *Curbside Consultation in Oculoplastics:*
49 Clinical Questions, Second Edition (pp 55-57).
© 2016 Taylor & Francis Group.

happen in isolation when a genetic process is the cause, but it can occur and needs to be considered when other workup is unrevealing.

Preliminary tests and questions as listed above will help to identify the more common causes of ptosis such as involutional (levator aponeurotic dehiscence) ptosis, mechanical ptosis, brow ptosis with secondary eyelid ptosis, and thyroid eye disease (pseudoptosis). Patients with myasthenia gravis causing ptosis will usually have variability on exam and often have positive rest or ice tests (application of ice to the more ptotic eyelid for 2 minutes; elevation of the eyelid by greater than 1 mm is considered a positive test). When the ptosis does not improve, and if there are extraocular movement problems without pupillary or sensory deficits, then an inherited disorder must be considered more seriously. Ocular myasthenia gravis (OMG) can reproduce these findings as well and may not be distinguishable on initial assessment.

Two classes of genetic syndromes to consider include mitochondrial disorders, typically chronic progressive external ophthalmoplegia (CPEO), and various forms of muscular dystrophy including myotonic dystrophy (MD) and oculopharyngeal muscular dystrophy (OPMD). Patients may not be aware of other family members who are affected by these specific disorders but often recognize similar symptoms in family members. CPEO and similar mitochondrial disorders are maternally inherited, so careful questioning about the status of maternal relatives should occur. Similarly, both MD and OPMD are autosomal dominant disorders, and affected family members may be known. There is also a rare form of autosomal recessive OPMD, but most clinicians need not consider this given its rarity.

CPEO and OPMD both tend to present after age 40, although CPEO patients may develop symptomatic ptosis at an earlier age. Despite having ocular motility problems that may be quite severe, most CPEO patients do not have diplopia, even if there is dysconjugate gaze. The reason for the lack of diplopia is not clear, but presence of double vision should make the clinician more suspicious for OMG mimicking CPEO. Both ptosis and ocular motility may be asymmetric in CPEO (Figure 10-1), but variability is not typically present, whereas it is a hallmark of OMG. In OPMD, ptosis may be quite severe, and patients may develop diplopia as well with EOM weakness and ocular misalignment. Nonetheless, motility problems are less common in OPMD with ptosis being the prominent feature. Patients may not report swallowing troubles, and they should be questioned carefully about gagging or choking symptoms. Myasthenia gravis with bulbar involvement must be considered in the differential diagnosis, but OPMD usually has a more insidious onset and progressive symptoms without diurnal variation. The autosomal dominant inheritance often results in similar symptoms in family members, but misdiagnosis of OPMD as bulbar MG can occur, and existence of familial myasthenia heightens suspicion for OPMD. Finally, MD type 1 patients may have significant ptosis as well, but unlike CPEO and OPMD, there are usually other systemic manifestations that establish the diagnosis.

Both CPEO and OPMD are relatively uncommon conditions. The precise prevalence of CPEO is difficult to determine because of phenotypic variation as well as the occurrence of CPEO plus syndromes, including Kearns-Sayre syndrome, in which possible cardiac conduction defects must be investigated to address potentially life-threatening arrhythmias. These patients also may have a retinitis pigmentosa type fundus picture. Many CPEO cases are associated with the m.3243A>G mutation. Not all carriers of the mutation will manifest disease, and thus there may not be a positive family history. A genetic diagnosis can be obtained by analysis of a muscle biopsy specimen, either from the levator or orbicularis muscle during ptosis surgery or skeletal muscle elsewhere. Characteristic electron microscopic changes also may be seen in the tissue. The overall incidence of OPMD is about 1:100,000, but it is 100 times more common in the French Canadian population and affects 1 in 600 persons of Bukharan Jewish ancestry. Because family history often is known, further testing may be unnecessary but can be obtained by blood testing for expansion of a trinucleotide repeat sequence in the PABPN1 gene.

Treatment of these disorders is symptomatic, as no medical treatment exists for the ocular problems. So-called mitochondrial cocktails consisting of nutritional supplements (coenzyme

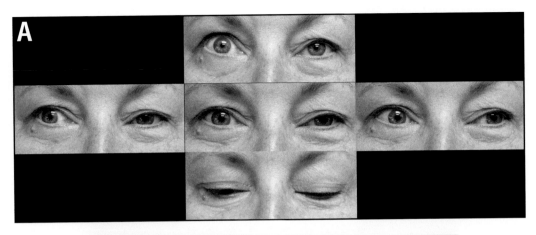

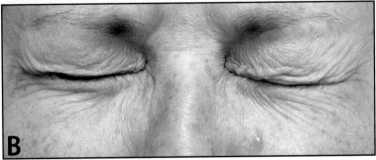

Figure 10-1. Motility and eyelid closure in CPEO. (A) Composite of eye movements in different positions of gaze showing asymmetric ptosis and marked limitation of all versions except downward. (B) Orbicularis oculi strength is normal and symmetric.

Q10, other antioxidants) have not shown long-term benefits. Ptosis surgery by levator resection or frontalis sling procedure may be performed, but strabismus surgery is rarely undertaken. Ptosis repair should be conservative because CPEO patients especially will have poor orbicularis muscle tone, increasing the risks for lagophthalmos and exposure keratopathy in the postoperative period. Both conditions are progressive over many years, although the pace of worsening is difficult to predict.

Suggested Readings

Allen RC, Zimmerman MB, Watterberg EA, Morrison LA, Carter KD. Primary bilateral silicone frontalis suspension for good levator function ptosis in oculopharyngeal muscular dystrophy. *Br J Ophthalmol.* 2012;96;841–845.

Fratter C, Gorman GS, Stewart JD, et al. The clinical, histochemical and molecular spectrum of PEO1 (Twinkle)-linked adPEO. *Neurology.* 2010;74;1619–1626.

Okulla T, Kunz WS, Klockgether T, Schröder R, Kornblum C. Diagnostic value of mitochondrial DNA mutation analysis in juvenile unilateral ptosis. *Graefes Arch Clin Exp.* 2005;243:380-382.

Soejima K, Sakurai H, Nozaki M, et al. Surgical treatment of blepharoptosis caused by chronic progressive external ophthalmoplegia. *Ann Plast Surg.* 2006;56:439-442.

WHY DOES AGE-RELATED BLEPHAROPTOSIS OCCUR?

Timothy J. McCulley, MD and
W. Jordan Piluek, MD

I've read that age-related blepharoptosis is the result of degeneration of the aponeurosis. I've noticed that when repairing ptotic eyelids, I often need to advance the aponeurosis to an abnormally low position. Could other factors be contributing? If so, what are the implications?

When patients present with acquired blepharoptosis, we often jump straight to treatment without giving much thought to cause. When patients ask, "What causes blepharoptosis?" we often answer with "old age" or "gravity." Sometimes we explain that the aponeurosis is stretched or disinserted. Surprisingly, this mechanism is not that well supported and may not (at least in some cases) be applicable. There are hundreds of conditions, not all benign, that may cause droopy eyelids. Question 9 addresses clues to when we should be worried about more significant disease. Here, we'll look at what causes involutional or age-related blepharoptosis. This insight will be helpful when counseling patients.

Evidence for degeneration of the aponeurosis consists of clinical and histopathological observations. In some elderly patients, elevation of the eyelid crease or simply the intraoperative observation of a flimsy aponeurosis suggests that in at least some cases, degeneration of the aponeurosis contributes to droopy eyelids (Figure 11-1). Also, blepharoptosis that occurs following placement of an eyelid speculum or with prolonged contact lens wear is well documented. In these cases, trauma to the aponeurosis is better established as the probable cause. Age-related ptosis appears and responds to surgery similarly, which could be used to argue for similar pathophysiology. Beyond these observations, there is little evidence to support this commonly assumed mechanism. Other than a few small, noncontrolled studies, careful histopathological evaluation of the aponeurosis and its contribution to eyelid ptosis has not been performed.

Sarcopenia is the term used to describe age-related loss of muscle mass and strength.[1] Suggested mechanisms include reductions in growth hormone and native anabolic steroid levels, increased catabolic cytokine levels, a decline in neural input, sedentary lifestyles, and dietary changes. There

Kersten RC, McCulley TJ, eds. *Curbside Consultation in Oculoplastics:
49 Clinical Questions, Second Edition* (pp 59-61).
© 2016 Taylor & Francis Group.

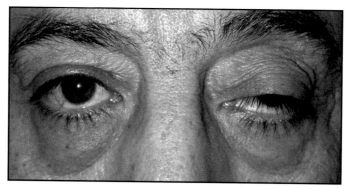

Figure 11-1. Acquired unilateral blepharoptosis. In this patient, the eyelid crease is elevated consistent with dehiscence of the levator aponeurosis.

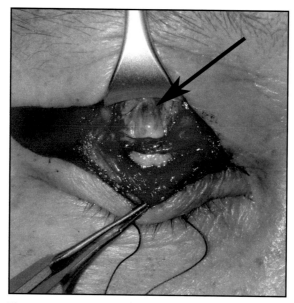

Figure 11-2. Intraoperative photo of levator superioris muscle with sarcopenia in a patient with acquired blepharoptosis. Fatty infiltration (arrow) is a hallmark of sarcopenia.

is no reason to believe that the levator superioris muscle would be spared. Several clinical observations indicate a muscular component to blepharoptosis, at least in a subgroup of patients. Patients with involutional blepharoptosis in whom complete advancement/resection of the aponeurosis fails to normalize the eyelid position are occasionally encountered. In such cases, if the muscle was fully functional, eyelid retraction would be expected. Commonly, fatty infiltration of the muscle is grossly evident (Figure 11-2). This fatty infiltration of muscles is a hallmark of sarcopenia. Moreover, there are a number of seemingly forgotten studies, which are rarely referenced, that described findings consistent with sarcopenia in patients with age-related blepharoptosis.[2,3] These qualitative changes in the microscopic appearance of the levator muscle are consistent with our notion that involutional muscular changes, at least in part, account for involutional eyelid ptosis.

In 2008, we contributed to a study looking at levator muscle health in patients with involutional blepharoptosis.[4] Although not to a degree to impact therapeutic or surgical approach, we found that the levator muscle strength (measured by eyelid excursion) was inversely proportional to degree of blepharoptosis. This is consistent with blepharoptosis being a component of sarcopenia.

Summary

Seemingly valid evidence for degeneration of both the levator superioris muscle and its aponeurosis exists. This evidence is not necessarily contradictory. It is likely that degeneration of both muscle and aponeurosis play contributory roles of varying degrees among individuals. Given our findings and those of the other investigators, it seems appropriate to consider acquired blepharoptosis the result of degenerative changes of both the levator superioris aponeurosis and the muscle itself. This explanation may be helpful when a patient inquires as to why their eyelids are starting to droop. Also, there is much effort currently going into looking at ways to prevent or even reverse age-related sarcopenia. It is probable that in the near future, we'll have medical therapy to manage age-related weakness. This may prove to be the future for management of eyelid ptosis.

References

1. Roubenoff R. Sarcopenia: a major modifiable cause of frailty in the elderly. *J Nutr Health Aging.* 2000;4:140-142.
2. Dortzback RK, Sutula FC. Involutional blepharoptosis: a histopathological study. *Arch Ophthalmol.* 1980;98:2045-2049.
3. Hornblass A, Adachi M, Wolintz A, Smith B. Clinical and ultrastructural correlation in congenital and acquired ptosis. *Ophthalmic Surg.* 1976;7:69-76.
4. Pereira LS, Hwang TN, Kersten RC, Ray K, McCulley TJ. Levator superioris muscle function in involutional blepharoptosis. *Am J Ophthalmol.* 2008;145:1095-1098.

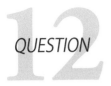

HOW SHOULD I MANAGE BLEPHAROPTOSIS?

Steven C. Dresner, MD

Please tell me more about managing blepharoptosis with a Müllerectomy. When should a transconjunctival (Müllerectomy or Fasanella-Servat) approach to blepharoptosis be used and when should a transcutaneous (levator advancement surgery) approach be used? Can a Müllerectomy be performed in the clinic?

Müllerectomy

A Müllerectomy is a quick, easy surgery in which Müller's muscle and underlying conjunctiva are excised. It is also known by such names as a posterior, transconjunctival, or internal blepharoptosis repair. It differs from the traditional Fasanella-Servat procedure in that none of the tarsus is excised. Although some clinicians still use the Fasanella-Servat procedure, there is a trend toward performing a Müllerectomy.

When evaluating any patient with blepharoptosis, I recommend that you perform a complete ophthalmic examination. Pay particular attention to the pupils, which may be abnormal with either a Horner syndrome or oculomotor nerve dysfunction. For similar reasons, pay particular attention to, and document, the extraocular motility. Any orbital asymmetry should be noted and exophthalmometry measurements recorded. Evaluate the conjunctival surface and note that any scarring or infiltrate in the superior fornix suggests an alternate cause of blepharoptosis and may require further evaluation.

There are several measures of eyelid height. I prefer the margin reflex distance-1 (MRD1), which is the distance between the corneal light reflex and the upper eyelid margin. Some document the margin reflex distance-2 (MRD2), which is the distance from the light reflex to the

Kersten RC, McCulley TJ, eds. *Curbside Consultation in Oculoplastics: 49 Clinical Questions, Second Edition* (pp 63-68).
© 2016 Taylor & Francis Group.

lower eyelid margin. The MRD1 and the MRD2 together should add up to the measurement of the palpebral fissure.

The levator excursion, also called levator function, should be tested on both sides. The levator excursion is measured by having the patient look down and then up with the brow stabilized. The excursion from extreme downgaze to upgaze estimates the levator muscle function and health. I consider poor function to be an excursion of less than 5 mm, fair function is 6 to 10 mm, and good function is anything over 10 mm. Patients with involutional blepharoptosis should have good function. If levator function is reduced, then look for an alternate etiology for the ptosis.

As part of a blepharoptosis evaluation, it is also important to note other involutional changes, such as brow ptosis, dermatochalasis, and lower eyelid and midface issues. Often, it is a combination of these factors that contribute to the patient's concerns. If neglected, even a patient with skillfully performed blepharoptosis repair might remain unhappy.

I like to photograph all of my patients to document the degree of blepharoptosis as well as other involutional changes. If you plan to bill the patient's insurance company, you will also want to perform visual field testing with the eyelids taped and untaped. This verifies the visual significance of the blepharoptosis.

Once I have completed the examination and have concluded that the patient has involutional blepharoptosis, the next step is to decide the best procedure to recommend. Specifically, would it be better to perform a levator advancement or a posterior blepharoptosis repair? There are many factors that influence this decision.

The severity of blepharoptosis, in part, dictates which procedure is best. Levator advancement surgery can be used to fix any degree of blepharoptosis, whereas a posterior approach is usually only able to correct blepharoptosis up to a maximum of 3 mm. Accordingly, involutional blepharoptosis of greater than 3 mm is best corrected with levator aponeurosis advancement through an external approach. In patients with mild blepharoptosis of 3 mm or less, a Müllerectomy can be considered. A phenylephrine test is used to determine whether or not a patient is even a candidate for a Müllerectomy.

There are many variations of the phenylephrine test. I like to perform the test by instilling 2 drops of 2.5% phenylephrine into the eye(s) with blepharoptosis. After 5 minutes, the MRD1 is again assessed. I consider a rise of the MRD1 of 2 mm or more to be a positive test. This indicates that a Müllerectomy procedure can be performed. It also gives the patient an idea of what can be expected from this type of surgery. If, with phenylephrine, the eyelid height remains low, this indicates that a Müller's muscle resection will not result in adequate eyelid elevation. For these patients, I usually recommend a Fasanella-Servat procedure if the ptosis is 2.5 mm, or less or a levator aponeurotic repair.

Whether or not I plan to perform a blepharoplasty also influences my decision. If the patient has elected to have a blepharoplasty in addition to blepharoptosis repair, I may lean toward a transcutaneous incision with levator advancement. This approach easily facilitates removal of excess skin and fat. It should be mentioned, however, that there are physicians who still prefer a Müllerectomy to levator advancement, even when performed in conjunction with a blepharoplasty. This eliminates the need for patient cooperation as required with levator surgery. Also, the orbicularis plane can be preserved. Some believe that this reduces the chance of postoperative lagophthalmos. Fat can still be removed through small buttonholes if desired.

Another consideration is anesthesia. Levator advancement surgery requires patient participation and often minimal discomfort is experienced. Performing levator advancement under straight local anesthesia can be done, but I would suggest selecting your patients carefully. Only offer this procedure to patients who will remain cooperative under anxious and slightly uncomfortable circumstances. Many patients are better served with monitored anesthesia. One of the great advantages of a Müllerectomy is that it can be performed under straight local anesthesia with no discomfort beyond that of the anesthetic injection. Patient participation is also not needed with a Müllerectomy, making it the preferred procedure for many patients.

The Müller's muscle resection procedure was introduced by Putterman and Urist.[1,2] Since its initial descriptions, many slight modifications have been suggested. The way I prefer to perform a Müllerectomy is illustrated in Figure 12-1. The amount of resection can be adjusted slightly to achieve small differences in the degree of elevation. I have found that usually 2 mm of blepharoptosis will require an 8-mm resection of Müller's muscle and conjunctiva. If I want slightly more elevation, I will excise up to 10 mm; if I want less than 2 mm elevation, I will excise less—down to about 6 mm.

Müllerectomy is a nice procedure for patients with involutional blepharoptosis and good levator function, who respond favorably on phenylephrine testing. It has the advantages of not requiring patient cooperation and it can easily be performed in the office under local anesthesia.

The Modified Fasanella-Servat Procedure

Small amounts of ptosis (1 to 2.5 mm) are treated with a Müeller's muscle conjunctival resection in the presence of a positive phenylephrine test. In patients with a negative phenylephrine test, a modified Fasanella-Servat procedure is very useful. This procedure is easy, quick, and predictable.

Preoperatively, an upper eyelid mark is placed above the pupillary axis, with the patient sitting upright (Figure 12-2A). A modified Müllerectomy clamp or a traditional Putterman clamp is used in this technique. Topical anesthetic drops are applied. The upper lid is anesthetized through the upper fornix with 1% lidocaine with epinephrine and hyaluronidase. The patient is prepped and draped for surgery. The eyelid is everted over a Desmarres retractor. Calipers are used to measure the proposed resection amount and the tarsus is marked centrally along the pupillary axis (Figure 12-2B). Two millimeters of tarsus is resected for each millimeter of desired correction. Two 4-0 silk sutures are placed through the tarsoconjunctival border medially and laterally for traction (Figure 12-2C). The retractor is removed and the tissues are elevated via the traction sutures. The clamp is placed over the tarsus and conjunctiva centered on the previously marked resection point (Figure 12-2D). The tissues are crushed with the clamp. A 6-0 Prolene suture is passed from the eyelid skin surface about 5 mm above the eyelid margin to the conjunctiva under the clamp (Figure 12-2E). The Prolene is then passed back and forth with 3 to 4 mm spacing in a horizontal running fashion 1 mm below the clamp and exiting through the skin at the other end of the clamp. The Prolene sutures are pulled firmly by the assistant and the clamped tissues are excised with a number 15 Bard-Parker blade, metal on metal of the clamp (Figure 12-2F). The eyelid is reflected back in its anatomic position and the suture is tied to itself in the pretarsal area (Figure 12-2G). No cautery is necessary. Ointment is applied to the area. The suture is removed in 5 to 7 days by cutting the external portion and pulling the remainder out.

The ratio of resection to the desired amount of correction is 2-to-1. The results are quite predictable (Figure 12-3). Complications include overcorrection, undercorrection, and possible contour abnormalities; however, overcorrection and contour problems are rare. Undercorrection usually requires subsequent levator repair. The modified Fasanella-Servat procedure is a useful adjunct to the ptosis surgeon's armamentarium of surgical techniques.

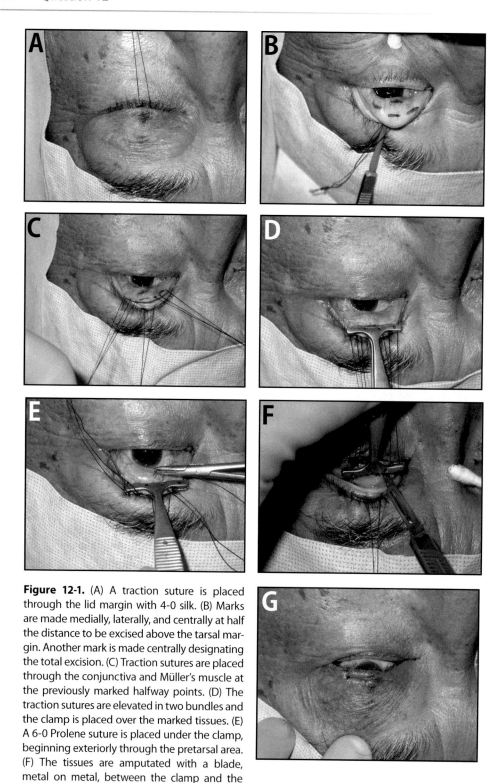

Figure 12-1. (A) A traction suture is placed through the lid margin with 4-0 silk. (B) Marks are made medially, laterally, and centrally at half the distance to be excised above the tarsal margin. Another mark is made centrally designating the total excision. (C) Traction sutures are placed through the conjunctiva and Müller's muscle at the previously marked halfway points. (D) The traction sutures are elevated in two bundles and the clamp is placed over the marked tissues. (E) A 6-0 Prolene suture is placed under the clamp, beginning exteriorly through the pretarsal area. (F) The tissues are amputated with a blade, metal on metal, between the clamp and the Prolene sutures. (G) The suture is exteriorized through the pretarsal area and sewn to itself. The lid margin traction suture is removed.

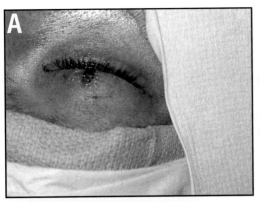

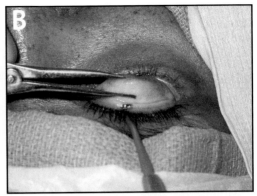

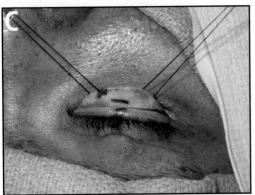

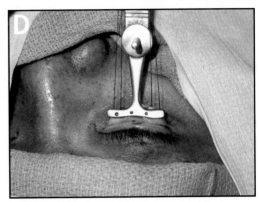

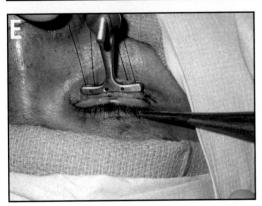

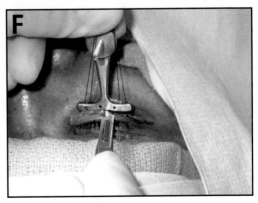

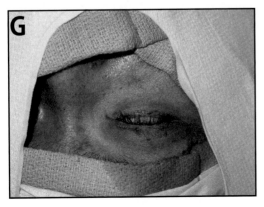

Figure 12-2. (A) An upper eyelid mark is placed above the pupillary axis. (B) A mark is made on the tarsus in the pupillary axis for the resection amount. (C) Traction sutures are placed medially and laterally on the upper tarsal edge. (D) The clamp is placed over the marked tissues. (E) A 6-0 Prolene suture is placed through the anterior lamella, under the clamp and out again. (F) The clamped tissues are excised, metal on metal. (G) The Prolene suture is tied over itself.

Figure 12-3. (A) Preoperative and (B) postoperative modified Fasanella-Servat procedure.

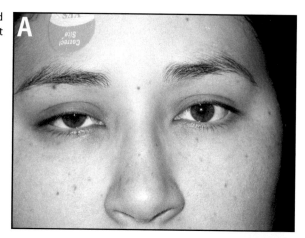

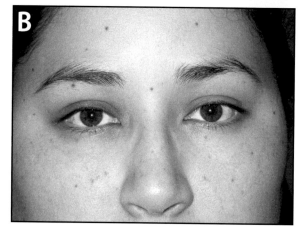

References

1. Putterman AM, Urist MJ. Müller muscle-conjunctiva resection. Technique for treatment of blepharoptosis. *Arch Ophthalmol.* 1975;93(8):619-623.
2. Dresner SC. Further modifications of the Muller's muscle-conjunctival resection procedure for blepharoptosis. *Ophthal Plast Reconstr Surg.* 1991;7:114-122.

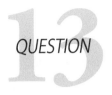

HOW DO I MANAGE A
CHILD WITH CONGENITAL BLEPHAROPTOSIS?

Maryam Nazemzadeh, MD; William R. Katowitz, MD; and
James A. Katowitz, MD

I'm fairly comfortable with acquired blepharoptosis and am considering helping children. How do you assess children with congenital blephaorptosis, and what do you think is the best surgical approach?

The management of pediatric ptosis continues to be challenging for ophthalmic surgeons. It requires an understanding of the innate anatomical differences between the adult and pediatric eyelid, including the differences in the mechanism of ptosis between these two patient populations. The timing of surgery and the specific technique have also proven to be challenging concepts. This chapter will outline the surgical approach and timing for the repair of pediatric ptosis.

Approach to Diagnosis

Determining the type of surgical technique and timing of surgery requires careful diagnosis in the pediatric setting. This begins with the determination of visual acuity. Presence of amblyopia or subnormal vision requires early intervention to allow proper development of the visual pathway. This may necessitate surgical intervention if more conservative measures are unlikely to be more effective. Formal visual acuity testing should be attempted whenever possible, but in children this may be difficult. One should always attempt to assess if a patient with congenital ptosis has preferential fixation with the non-ptotic eye because this suggests the development of amblyopia.

Assessing the severity of ptosis is best done by measuring the margin-reflex distance MRD1 (distance of the central upper eyelid margin to the center of the pupillary light reflex). In cases of unilateral ptosis, a higher brow position on the affected side is a clue that the frontalis muscle is being recruited to raise the eyelid above the pupillary axis. This is reassuring to note because it indicates that the patient continues to prefer single binocular vision and has not yet begun to

Kersten RC, McCulley TJ, eds. *Curbside Consultation in Oculoplastics:
49 Clinical Questions, Second Edition* (pp 69-74).
© 2016 Taylor & Francis Group.

Figure 13-1. (A) One-year-old child with a left congenital ptosis. (B) Elevation of the left upper lid to symmetrical position following one drop of 2.5% phenylephrine. (C) Six-month postoperative result following modified Fasanella-Servat tarso-Müllerectomy.

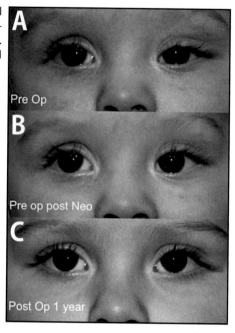

develop amblyopia. A chin-up position is another adaptive technique that children use to clear their pupillary axis. The absence of these subtle clues should raise the alarm for amblyopia and the assistance of a pediatric ophthalmologist is often important.

The degree of levator function in relation to the amount of ptosis is an important factor in surgical planning. This is done with the child looking up and down while stabilizing the frontalis muscle. Poor levator function or a levator excursion of less than 3 to 5 mm often requires the use of an alternate anatomical structure to lift the lid. Our preference is to use frontalis suspension because of corneal complications frequently associated with the use of the superior rectus for lid elevation. Levator function of greater than 5 to 6 mm indicates that surgical strengthening of some aspect of the retractor mechanism within the eyelid. The structures involved include the tarsus, Müller's muscle, levator muscle, and the levator aponeurosis. To determine the specific retraction mechanism that should be targeted during surgery, the surgeon should quantify the patient's response to one topical drop of 2.5% phenylephrine (Figure 13-1). The drop targets Müller's sympathetic muscle and a positive response indicates that a Müller's muscle resection (with or without tarsectomy) will usually produce a similar postoperative result. The use of this drop can also unmask ptosis on the seemingly normal eyelid. If the ptotic eyelid responds to phenylephrine and the opposite eyelid drops, then one has unmasked a contralateral ptosis. This response is due to Hering's law, which states that equal and simultaneous innervation flows to synergistic muscles.[1] The phenylephrine response reduces the extra effort that was previously placed on the affected side and therefore energy to the opposite levator muscle, or the contralateral yoke muscle, is also reduced.

Surgical Approaches

Ptosis surgery can be completed either through an anterior (external) or posterior (internal) approach. Internal procedures include the conjunctivo-Müllerectomy (Putterman), tarso-conjunctivo Müllerectomy (Fasanella-Servat), and the Müller-levator muscle resection (Werb) procedures. The underlying mechanism of these procedures is strengthening the retraction system within the eyelid. Internal approaches for shortening Müller's muscle are particularly effective if the child demonstrates a good response to topical phenylephrine. The major advantage to these procedures is that they offer relatively predictable postoperative outcomes because they mimic stimulation of Müller's muscle with topical phenylephrine. This becomes especially useful in the pediatric setting because it gives parents a good estimation as to where the eyelid will sit post-operatively as well as identifying cases of masked ptosis on the contralateral side. In addition, because general anesthesia is used for these pediatric cases, intraoperative adjustments cannot be performed, further demonstrating the advantage of the predictability of these procedures. Another advantage is the minimal postoperative lagophthalmos. Poor response to phenylephrine indicates the need for levator surgery or a frontalis suspension procedure.

INTERNAL APPROACHES

The Fasanella-Servat procedure (tarsoconjunctival Müllerectomy) involves resection of the upper tarsus, Müller's muscle, and the overlying conjunctiva. This procedure is usually recommended in patients with mild ptosis (3 mm or less) and good levator function.[2] However, this procedure can be used with higher degrees of ptosis in patients with a good response to phenylephrine.

The traditional Fasanella-Servat procedure begins with the eversion of the upper eyelid to treat the posterior or internal aspect of the eyelid. Two curved hemostats are used to clamp and isolate the Müller's muscle between the superior tarsus and the overlying conjunctiva. The amount of tissue clamped directly correlates with the amount of correction or lift that is desired. The surgeon must remember to leave behind at least 5 mm of tarsus to prevent destabilization of the eyelid. This will prevent the occurrence of an upper eyelid entropion. The two hemostats are maintained while a double-armed catgut suture is passed below the clamp in a running fashion. The tissue is then resected below the clamps but above the suture, and the second arm of the suture is used to approximate the wound edges.[3]

At the Children's Hospital of Philadelphia (CHOP), we use a modified version of the Fasanella-Servat, which includes stabilizing the upper eyelid after clamp placement with two 4-0 black silk sutures placed medially and laterally. The clamps are then removed, and the tissue is resected above the crush marks. Then a running 5-0 nylon suture is passed in a subcuticular fashion with 4 or 5 bites in the undersurface of tarsus and Müller's muscle. The inner lining of the conjunctiva is included in the bites to prevent retraction. With this technique, Müller's muscle can be further advanced by including more muscle in the passes with the suture. The incorporation of more Müller's muscle can give an overcorrection compared to the amount of preoperative lift given by the topical phenylephrine. This is useful in patients who have a good response to phenylephrine and good levator function, but require a mild amount of additional lift (see Figure 13-1).

The Putterman procedure (conjunctivo-Müllerectomy) is another internal approach that targets the Müller's muscle, although this technique spares the tarsus. The Werb procedure (Müller-levator muscle resection) is an internal technique that incorporates both the Müller and levator muscles. Surgeons may find this more difficult than an external levator approach because the surgeon must navigate through the upper eyelid anatomy from an upside down position. Also, this procedure does not permit simple levator aponeurosis advancement as easily, which may be necessary in certain situations.

EXTERNAL APPROACHES

The levator aponeurosis advancement and levator resection procedures are most easily completed via an external or anterior approach. At CHOP, we prefer to follow Berke's principles and position the eyelid relative to the superior corneal limbus depending on the preoperative measurements of the levator function.[4] Based on Berke's concepts, the amount of resection to be performed

Table 13-1
Intraoperative Eyelid Height

Upper Eyelide Excursion	Superior Corneal Coverage by Upper Eyelid
0 to 5 mm (poor)	0 mm (lid margin at superior limbus)
6 to 11 mm (fair)	2 mm
12 mm or more (good)	4 mm

is determined by setting the position of the lid level relative to the superior corneal limbus at the time of surgery with the patient under general anesthesia (Table 13-1).[5,6]

We base this decision on the strength of the levator muscle and its elasticity. In general, it is advisable to overcorrect congenital myogenic ptosis and to undercorrect acquired ptosis. The weaker the levator function, the greater the overcorrection required, as the lid will drop in the postoperative period. If levator function is poor, an overcorrection of 2 mm is advisable. If levator function is fair, 1 mm of overcorrection is recommended. For those cases of ptosis with good levator function, the lid should be set 2 to 3 mm below the superior corneal limbus because the postoperative force of the levator contraction will be more effective. Likewise, for excellent levator function, the lid placement should be 3 to 4 mm below the superior corneal limbus.

External levator surgery requires a lid crease incision to gain access to the upper eyelid anatomy. Once the lid crease incision is complete, the septum is dissected through until preaponeurotic fat is encountered. The levator muscle and its aponeurosis are isolated. In the case of the levator aponeurosis advancement, the aponeurosis is undermined from Müller's muscle below and reattached or advanced onto the tarsus with 5-0 Vicryl sutures. Three double-armed 5-0 Vicryl sutures are placed partial thickness through the tarsus then through the levator. The sutures should be placed in a mattress fashion no more than one-third below the superior margin to avoid eversion of the eyelid. The first suture is placed in a position halfway between the center of the pupil and the medial limbus. The remaining two are placed medially and laterally in relation to the first.[7]

Levator resection is done by creating two buttonhole incisions with closed scissors above the tarsus through the levator muscle, Müller's muscle, and the conjunctiva medially and laterally. A Berke ptosis clamp is guided through the buttonholes with the scissors. The clamp is then closed and includes the levator muscle, Müller's muscle, and conjunctiva. The tissue between the clamp and the superior border of the tarsus is severed. The tissue in the clamp is everted to reveal the underlying conjunctiva. Scissors are used to dissect the plane between the conjunctiva and Müller's muscle. It is best to enter the conjunctiva 10 to 12 mm above the tarsus where there is a surgical plane for dissection. The scissors are used to carefully spread the conjunctiva away from the underlying Müller's muscle. About 4 to 5 mm of conjunctiva is resected to minimize the chance of postoperative prolapse. No adverse effects on the tear film have been noted objectively or subjectively in our experience with this conjunctival resection. The remaining conjunctiva is reapproximated to the superior tarsal border with interrupted 6-0 plain catgut sutures. Then three 5-0 Vicryl mattress sutures are passed between the tarsus and levator muscle as described previously. The sutures are first temporarily tied with a bow-knot to ensure proper lid height and contour. Once this is established, the surgeon permanently ties the sutures down. Excess levator and Müller's muscle is excised. Finally, one end of each suture is passed through the subcutaneous tissue of the inferior skin edge of the skin incision and tied to the knot in the levator muscle to recreate the lid crease and fold. Skin should be judiciously removed to allow for the looser superior preseptal skin and orbicularis to gently fold over the lid crease. The skin incision can be closed with a running 6-0 fast-absorbing catgut suture.

In general, care is taken not to cut or violate Whitnall's ligament, particularly in the setting of extensive resection. In general, we recommend avoiding cutting the levator horns because significant elasticity is lost even in dystrophic muscles. In certain instances, however, this cannot be avoided, as sufficient lid lift is impossible without cutting the horns.

FRONTALIS SUSPENSION

In patients with poor levator function, the procedure of choice is frontalis suspension. The use of autogenous fascia lata is reserved for children aged 4 to 5 years and older, when the leg is of sufficient length to harvest the graft.

Synthetic materials and donor tissue have been used due to the morbidity associated with harvesting autogenous material in younger children. With the use of donor tissue, careful patient selection and gamma irradiation of cadaveric donor fascia are imperative in reducing the risk for infection, but even with this, the elimination of prions is debated. However, the use of donor tissue has its drawbacks. The long-term success rates and recurrence of ptosis in previous studies has caused its use to be questioned.[8] We prefer the use of synthetic materials in children younger than 4 years and prefer silicone slings due to the lower rate of complications and failure. The material is easy to place and is rarely associated with granuloma formation or infection.[9] Other materials that can be used for frontalis sling include 4-0 Prolene sutures, Goretex sutures, or marlex mesh.

Timing of Surgery

As discussed earlier, the timing of surgery in the pediatric population is extremely important. In cases of occlusion or anisometropic amblyopia, surgery is done as early as possible to allow the proper development of vision. If there is no evidence of amblyopia, we prefer surgery to be performed at 1 year of age. Our rationale for early surgery is based on several factors:

- There is no additional anesthetic risk to the child after 6 months of age
- The emotional stress on the child and family may be reduced if surgery is performed at a younger age
- The lid structures are adequate in size
- Our surgical outcomes in the younger age group appear to be as good as the results in older children

Summary

Our recommendations for repair of childhood ptosis are to plan the surgery based on the response to topical phenylephrine (Table 13-2). If the response to phenylephrine is inadequate but there is reasonable levator function, then some form of levator surgery should be performed. One should reserve frontalis suspension for ptosis with fair to poor levator function (Table 13-3). Synthetic materials are useful in patients younger than 4 years. Autogenous fascia lata is preferred for older children.

Table 13-2
Selection of Ptosis Based on the Response to Phenylephrine

Response to Phenylephrine	Surgical Procedure
Good (MRD1 = 4 to 5)	Putterman Müllerectomy or modified Fasanella-Servat
Moderate (MRD1 = 3)	Graded modified Fasanell-Servat or Werb procedure (ie, graded Müllerectomy with tarsectomy)
Poor (MRDI ≤2)	Levator surgery or frontalis suspension

The degree of preop levator function is not critical in procedure selection if response is good to moderate.
Reprinted with permission from Heher KL, Katowitz JA. Pediatric ptosis. In: Katowitz JA, ed. *Pediatric Oculoplastic Surgery.* New York, NY: Springer-Verlag; 2002: 253-288. © 2002 Springer Science+Business Media.

Table 13-3
Classification of Levator Function

Levator Function	Eyelid Excursion
Excellent	≥13 mm
Good	8 to 12 mm
Fair	5 to 7 mm
Poor	≤4 mm

References

1. Wright KW, Spiegal PH. *Pediatric Ophthalmology and Strabismus.* St. Louis, MO: CV Mosby; 1999:149-166
2. Collin JR. *A Manual of Systemic Eyelid Surgery.* Edinburgh: Churchill Livingstone; 1989.
3. Fasanella RM, Servat J. Levator resection for minimal ptosis: another simplified operation. *Arch Ophthalmol.* 1961;65:493-496.
4. Berke RN. Surgical treatment of congenital ptosis. *Pac Med Surg.* 1967;75(6):383-388.
5. Berke RN. Results of resection of the levator muscle through a skin incision in congenital ptosis. *AMA Arch Ophthalmol.* 1959;61(2):177-201.
6. Berke RN. The surgical correction of congenital ptosis. *Trans Pa Acad Ophthalmol Otolaryngol.* 1961;14:57-61.
7. Heher KL, Katowitz JA. Pediatric ptosis. In Katowitz JA, ed. *Pediatric Oculoplastic Surgery.* New York, NY: Springer-Verlag; 2002:262-280.
8. Esmaeli B, Chung H, Pashby RC. Long-term results of frontalis suspension using irradiated, banked fascia lata. *Ophthalmic Plast Reconstr Surg.* 1998;14(3):159-163.
9. Katowitz J. Frontalis suspension in congenital ptosis using a polyfilament, cable-type suture. *Arch Ophthalmol.* 1979;97:1659-1663.

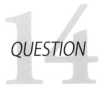

How Should I Manage Ectropion?

Daniel J. Townsend, MD

What is the appropriate evaluation of a patient with ectropion? How do you decide which surgical procedure will work best? What can be done to make the patient more comfortable while waiting for surgery?

Ectropion, or the turning out of the lower eyelid, is a common problem in the elderly population. Patients often complain of irritation and foreign body sensation due to exposure and drying of the ocular surface. Tearing is also a common complaint. The most common cause of ectropion is simply laxity of the eyelid. Lateral canthal tendon laxity is almost always present and, if associated with disinsertion of the inferior lid retractors, may result in complete eversion of the tarsal plate (ie, tarsus inversus). In severe cases, keratinization and fibrosis of the tarsal conjunctiva may occur. Other factors that should not be overlooked include scarring or shortening of the eyelid skin. Axial projection of the globe may also be a contributing factor. Identification of all contributing factors is essential in planning surgery.

Evaluation is directed toward determining if there is significant horizontal laxity of the eyelid, as well as whether there is vertical foreshortening of the anterior lamella. Patients should be asked about prior trauma or surgical intervention and any history of skin cancer of the head and neck region. Distraction of the eyelid and the snap-back test will demonstrate horizontal laxity. Visual examination and palpation of the lower eyelid skin may demonstrate cicatricial tightening or thickening. I always closely examine the lower eyelid skin in patients with cicatricial ectropion, looking for telangiectasias or ulceration that may suggest an underlying, unsuspected epithelial malignancy. Palpation of the skin is also helpful. If it feels firm, irregular, or thickened, this may suggest an unsuspected morpheaform basal cell carcinoma. When in doubt, I always obtain a punch biopsy of any suspicious area.

Patients with ectropion often experience epiphora, which can occur due to a number of factors. Ocular irritation may cause reactive tearing. Epiphora may also be due to eversion of the inferior

Kersten RC, McCulley TJ, eds. *Curbside Consultation in Oculoplastics: 49 Clinical Questions, Second Edition* (pp 75-77).
© 2016 Taylor & Francis Group.

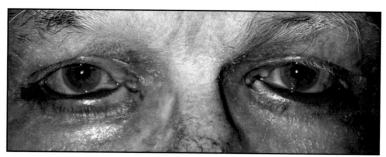

Figure 14-1. Bilateral ectropion due to horizontal laxity as well as actinic cicatricial changes.

puncta. A poorly functioning lacrimal pump, often the result of excess horizontal lid laxity, may also exacerbate the epiphora. However, I find that mild ectropion rarely causes very symptomatic tearing and before attributing epiphora to ectropion, it is imperative to examine the entire tear outflow system. One often finds that tearing may have initially started due to stenosis of the nasolacrimal duct, and that eversion or eyelid laxity may have occurred secondarily. Frequent wiping of the eyelids, which is occurring in response to the buildup of tears over the lower eyelid, may be the cause of laxity. Moreover, irritation from the overflowing tears themselves can cause induration and loss of elasticity of the eyelid skin, which also contributes to the malposition. In this case, ectropion repair must be accompanied by dacryocystorhinostomy to correct the underlying etiology.

The treatment for ectropion is surgical and must be based on the exact etiology of the eyelid malposition. Excess laxity needs to be addressed with horizontal shortening of the eyelid. A cicatricial ectropion with foreshortened or contracted skin may require augmentation of the anterior lamella, either through skin grafting or soft tissue transposition. Punctal malposition needs to be evaluated as well. Simple eversion of the punctum without accompanying eyelid laxity may be corrected by a spindle-shaped excision of conjunctiva and lower eyelid retractors. Often, several procedures are combined to fully repair an ectropion. I find that one of the most common reasons for recurrent ectropion following a surgical repair is failure to recognize or address cicatricial eyelid changes. Actinic damage alone may result in shortening of the eyelid skin to a degree sufficient to cause ectropion and is commonly overlooked (Figure 14-1).

Correction of ectropion usually involves addressing horizontal laxity. Even in primarily cicatricial ectropion, tightening of the eyelid is usually helpful. This is best done by a lateral tarsal strip–type of procedure, where the lateral tarsus is resuspended from the periosteum at the lateral orbital rim. Figure 14-2 shows this commonly performed tarsal strip procedure for repair of the horizontal laxity present to a greater or lesser degree in most cases of ectropion.

If there is coexisting vertical shortage of skin because of actinic changes, previous trauma, or surgery, then augmentation of the skin is usually also performed. Full-thickness skin grafts, usually harvested from the hairless pre- or retro-auricular areas, are usually preferred. Upper eyelid skin can be used but has thinner dermis and provides less support. Alternately, an upper to lower pedicle flap of skin and muscle can be used to augment the anterior lamella.

Summary

Involutional ectropion is a common eyelid malposition caused by tissue relaxation, dehiscence of canthal tendons, and laxity of lower eyelid retractors. In patients with ectropion and the primary

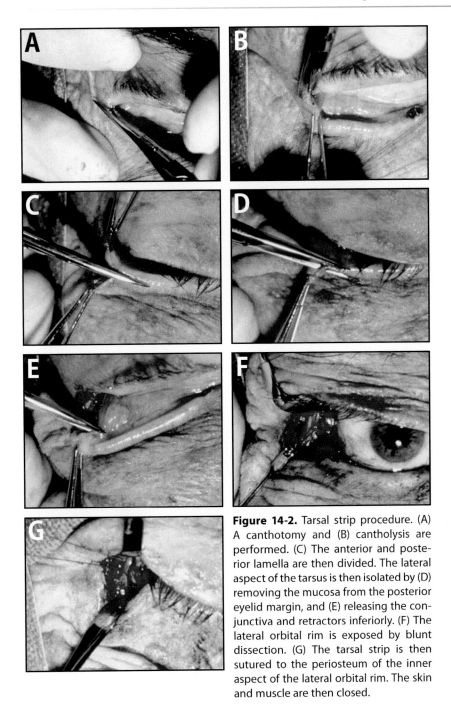

Figure 14-2. Tarsal strip procedure. (A) A canthotomy and (B) cantholysis are performed. (C) The anterior and posterior lamella are then divided. The lateral aspect of the tarsus is then isolated by (D) removing the mucosa from the posterior eyelid margin, and (E) releasing the conjunctiva and retractors inferiorly. (F) The lateral orbital rim is exposed by blunt dissection. (G) The tarsal strip is then sutured to the periosteum of the inner aspect of the lateral orbital rim. The skin and muscle are then closed.

complaint of epiphora, be sure to consider underlying nasolacrimal duct obstruction. Corrective surgical procedures typically involve a lateral tarsal strip tightening of the lax eyelid. Failure to address cicatricial eyelid changes is probably the most common cause for recurrence following a tarsal strip procedure.

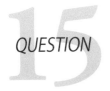
HOW DOES TRANSCONJUNCTIVAL LOWER EYELID ENTROPION REPAIR COMPARE WITH A TRANSCUTANEOUS APPROACH?

Catherine J. Hwang, MD and
Payam V. Morgan, MD

I recently attended an oculoplastics workshop and one of the instructors was suggesting an "internal" or conjunctival approach to entropion repair. Have you heard of this? Is this something I should be offering my patients?

There have been numerous publications on entropion surgery dating back to 1887.[1] The surgical approach for the correction of entropion has undergone numerous modifications over time. In the late 1800s, the main approach was to split the lid with or without taking a wedge of tarsus, which is still done today.[1,2] Since then, various techniques have been used to address involutional entropion: skin and subcutaneous tissue contraction by means of acid or application of cautery, removal of a triangle of skin from the zygomatic region to induce lateral traction on the skin of the lower eyelid, and weakening of the orbicularis by injection of 80% alcohol.[2,3] In addition, orbicularis transposition to the lateral orbital rim to provide traction laterally and weakening of the orbicularis became popular.[2,4]

When thinking about lower eyelid entropion surgery, one has to think about the mechanisms causing the entropion. Patients with involutional entropion have both horizontal lid laxity and disinsertion of the lower eyelid retractors. Addressing these anatomic changes will help guide successful surgery.

Both transcutaneous and transconjunctival approaches have been described; there are advantages and disadvantages to each. Both techniques rely on addressing the horizontal lid laxity and reinsertion of the lower eyelid retractors (the capsule-palpebral ligament). Horizontal lid laxity can been addressed with either a small-incision lateral canthal resuspension for mild to moderate lid laxity or a lateral tarsal strip for more severe laxity.[5] Reinsertion of the retractors can be done either through an anterior transcutaneous approach or posteriorly through a transconjunctival approach. A customized approach to each patient is key.

For those patients who have a more severe spastic entropion, a transcutaneous approach can be considered. A transcutaneous approach affords a better scar adhesion anteriorly and potentially less

Kersten RC, McCulley TJ, eds. *Curbside Consultation in Oculoplastics:*
49 Clinical Questions, Second Edition (pp 79-81).
© 2016 Taylor & Francis Group.

risk for recurrence of the entropion. A potential disadvantage to this surgery would be overcorrection and resultant ectropion, but anatomic placement of the eyelid without frank ectropion at the time of surgery should prevent this. The transcutaneous approach can be further customized and performed either through 3 small subciliary stab incisions or through a longer subciliary incision with removal of orbicularis and/or skin.[5] For patients with more of a spastic component, a longer subciliary incision may be more beneficial to allow for resection of a small strip of preseptal orbicularis and/or skin.

Although percutaneous incisions in the lower eyelid crease are virtually imperceptible, in those patients who are overly concerned about scarring (such as a pigmented or cosmetically-oriented patient), a transconjunctival approach may be used. The principles are the same with reinsertion of the retractors but the scar is on the posterior lamellae, which is well hidden. Removal of a small strip of preseptal orbicularis can also be performed combined with a horizontal tightening procedure, typically a tarsal strip.[6] Erb et al has reported a 3.3% recurrence rate after the transconjunctival approach for involutional entropion.[7]

Comparing the success of transcutaneous and transconjunctival approaches is not straight forward. Ben-Simon et al reported the recurrence rate to be slightly higher with a transconjunctival approach, but this was not statistically significant.[8] This study did not, however, remove orbicularis during the transconjunctival approach as described by Dresner et al.[6]

Ultimately, the surgeon must remember to be a problem solver and not just be a "procedure surgeon." Each patient who presents to us is unique and each surgery should be tailored to the patient. Involutional entropion surgery, either by transcutaneous or transconjunctival approaches, is successful as long as the anatomic issues of horizontal lid laxity and lower eyelid retractor disinsertion are addressed.

Surgical Technique

TRANSCUTANEOUS APPROACH

After proper anesthesia, 3 stab incisions or a single long incision is made in the subciliary space through skin and orbicularis.[8] Blunt dissection is then performed to reveal the lower eyelid retractors. The white edge of the lower eyelid retractors is then advanced to the anterior inferior border of the tarsal edge using 2 to 3 interrupted 5-0 polyglactin sutures. A small strip of presep-tal orbicularis and/or skin can then be removed prior to closure of the skin incision. With the small-incision technique, a small pocket is made to roughen the edge of the retractors centrally, medially, and laterally. The lower eyelid retractors are advanced by placing the polyglactin suture from the stab incision to the conjunctiva, engaging the lower eyelid retractors, back through the conjunctiva, and then securing the retractors to the anterior inferior tarsus. A horizontal tightening procedure is also performed by a small-incision canthoplasty or tarsal strip, depending on the degree of horizontal laxity.

TRANSCONJUNCTIVAL APPROACH

After proper anesthesia, a lateral canthotomy is performed and the inferior crus of the lateral canthal tendon is severed.[6] A transconjuctival incision is made from the lateral canthotomy site to the punctum just below the inferior border of tarsus. The surgical plane is carried down toward the orbital rim between the septum and retractors. The lower eyelid is then everted and a small strip of orbicularis muscle is excised. Next, the retractors are separated from the conjunctiva to form a free edge and then reinserted to the anterior inferior border of the tarsus with 2 buried 5-0 polyglactin sutures. The conjunctiva is not sutured. Horizontal tightening is performed with a lateral tarsal strip. The skin of the canthotomy site is then closed.

References

1. Benson AH. The operative treatment of trichiasis with or without entropion, and a short note on Argyll Robertson's operation for ectropion. *Br Med J.* 1887;1(1378):1154-1156.
2. MacRae A. Webster's operation for entropion of the upper lid. *J Ophthalmol.* 1928;12(1):25-30.
3. Sorsby A. Spasmodic entropion treated by injection of alcohol. *Proc R Soc Med.* 1931;24(5):611.
4. Wheeler JM. Spastic entropion correction by orbicularis transplantation. *Trans Am Ophthalmol Soc.* 1938;36:157-162.
5. Taban M, Nakra T, Hwang C, et al. Aesthetic lateral canthoplasty. *Ophthal Plast Reconstr Surg.* 2010;26(3):190-194.
6. Dresner SC, Karesh JW. Transconjunctival entropion repair. *Arch Ophthalmol.* 1993;111(8):1144-1148.
7. Erb MH, Uzcategui N, Dresner SC. Efficacy and complications of the transconjunctival entropion repair for lower eyelid involutional entropion. *Ophthalmology.* 2006;113(12):2351-2356.
8. Ben Simon GJ, Molina M, Schwarcz RM, McCann JD, Goldberg RA. External (subciliary) vs internal (transconjunctival) involutional entropion repair. *Am J Ophthalmol.* 2005;139(3):482-487.

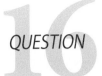

WHAT IS THE ROLE OF TARSORRHAPHY?

Gary L. Aguilar, MD and
Robert C. Kersten, MD, FACS

When would you suggest a temporary tarsorrhaphy? When would you recommend a permanent tarsorrhaphy? What techniques would you suggest for both?

In the ophthalmologist's surgical armamentarium, there are few procedures that are as important and useful as the one used to close the eyelids—surgical tarsorrhaphy. Conditions that call for the procedure are those that threaten corneal injury, which fall into 2 main categories: (1) exposure keratopathy due to lagophthalmos, or (2) primary corneal dysfunction. Exposure may be due to a number of causes but most often relates to facial nerve dysfunction. Other common causes include exophthalmos and eyelid retraction. Quite a number of corneal problems are best treated by closing the eyelids, if only temporarily. In a study that examined a cohort of corneal and external disease patients who had undergone tarsorrhaphy, indications for the surgery included neurotrophic ulcers, penetrating keratoplasty-related epithelial problems, postinfection epithelial problems, severe dry eye syndrome, radiation keratopathy, ocular cicatricial pemphigoid, and Stevens-Johnson syndrome.[1]

Depending on the indications for the procedure, tarsorrhaphy may be permanent or temporary. In addition, if there is a need for regular evaluation of the underlying ocular surface, a pillar tarsorraphy will allow distraction of the apposed eyelids for purposes of examination. Temporary tarsorrhaphies are easily performed, may be left in place for several weeks at a time, and can dramatically improve corneal pathology. They are useful as a temporizing measure when immediate protection of the cornea is needed, while plans for definitive treatment are made (eg, a patient with facial nerve paralysis who is waiting for a scheduled gold weight placement). We also use temporary tarsorrhaphies in the immediate postoperative period following such procedures as placement of a skin graft, repair of a lower eyelid retraction, and following enucleation. Permanent tarsorrhaphies

Kersten RC, McCulley TJ, eds. *Curbside Consultation in Oculoplastics:*
49 Clinical Questions, Second Edition (pp 83-87).
© 2016 Taylor & Francis Group.

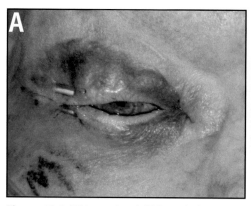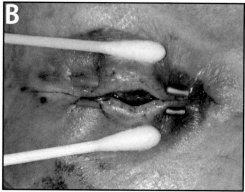

Figure 16-1. (A) Lateral and (B) lateral plus medial tarsorrhaphy.

are reserved for patients with long-standing corneal pathology (eg, neurotrophic keratitis) where less disfiguring procedures are not effective.

Another consideration is how much of the eye to close. Generally, it is the lateral lid margins that are conjoined, but when greater corneal coverage is needed, lid closure may be performed both laterally and medially (Figure 16-1).

A larger variety of techniques have been described and advocated. We will run through some of the more common ones.

Glue Tarsorrhaphy

In 1966, Schimek and Ballou[2] first described a sutureless technique in which the eyelids were glued together by means of a temporary adhesive—cyanoacrylate liquid. This will usually result in apposition of the eyelids for 5 to 7 days and can be repeated. One must take care to avoid inadvertent spillage of the glue leading to unpredictable amounts of eyelid adhesion, or corneal irritation.

Suture Tarsorrhaphy

Temporary tarsorrhaphy involves suturing of the apposing eyelid margins together. To allow precise apposition, the sutures at the lid margin need to pass through the tarsal plate in a mirror image of upper and lower eyelids. The Meibomian gland orifices provide a good guide to the center of the tarsal plate and we prefer to pass the needle directly through these to ensure exact approximation. We generally prefer to pass the suture in a lamellar fashion within the tarsus of the upper and lower eyelid, entering and exiting the needle through the lid margin (see Figure 16-1), so that the suture is visible only at the lid margin. This obviates the need for bolsters or exposure of suture ends. It is important to use a half-circle needle to ensure that the lamellar pass through tarsus is deep enough to prevent cheese-wiring of the suture through the tarsus, which will result in separation of the lids or complete dehiscence of the apposition.

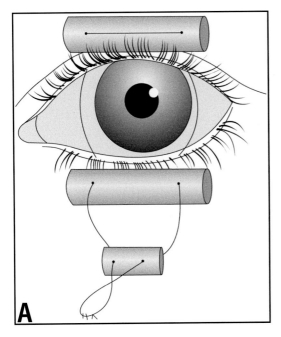

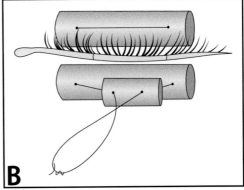

Figure 16-2. Drawstring temporary tarsorrhaphy. (A) Sutures are passed through large bolsters and (B) tied using a slip knot. The suture tails are long enough for loosening and retying, if necessary.

Drawstring Tarsorrhaphy

A useful modification of the suture method is the so-called drawstring, temporary tarsorrhaphy technique.[3] With this technique, the lids can be closed, opened, and closed again as needed to inspect the anterior segment. Double-armed, 5-0 Prolene sutures are passed through sections of a rubber Foley catheter and then through the skin and orbicularis 4 mm proximal to the eyelid margin, exiting through the Meibomian gland orifices in a mirror-image fashion in the upper and lower eyelids. The sutures are then tied with a slip knot, which can be tied and untied to allow opening of the lids (Figure 16-2).

Permanent Tarsorrhaphy

We use a similar suture placement whether performing a permanent or temporary tarsorrhaphy. The only difference is that permanent tarsorraphy involves denuding the mucocutaneous epithelium overlying the tarsal plate at the eyelid margin prior to passing appositional sutures. It is important that excision of the epithelium remain superficial and not extend into the underlying tarsus to allow future takedown of the tarsorraphy without concern for development of an eyelid margin notch or cicatricial entropion and trichiasis. The epithelium over the tarsal plate (posterior aspect of the lid margin behind the grey line), can either be shaved with a number 11 Bard-Parker blade or excised with Wescott scissors. If apposition of the lateral one-third of the tarsus is desired, We use a double-armed 5-0 Vicryl suture passed directly through the medial cut edge of the upper lid and directed well into the tarsus. The needle pass remains in the plane of the tarsus, exiting

Figure 16-3. Permanent tarsorrhaphy. The posterior edge of the opposing eyelid margins is de-epithelialized, taking care not to injure the underlying tarsal plate. A suture is passed through the cut edges of upper and lower eyelids. The sutures are tied with the knot buried. Alternatively, the suture can be passed through the eyelid margin of tarsus, exiting through orbicularis and skin anteriorly and tied over a bolster.

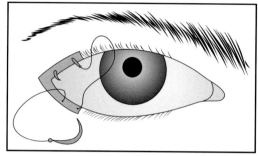

from the lateral edge of the upper eyelid. The opposing arm of the suture is then passed in a mirror-image fashion in the lower eyelid, entering medially and exiting laterally. The two suture ends are tied, bringing the denuded surfaces of the tarsal plates of the aposing eyelids together where they become adherent. If adherence of more than one-third of the aperture is desired, we use a 5-0 Prolene suture on a half-round needle, and begin passing through a bolster medially, entering skin 4 mm proximal to the eyelid margin, and exiting through the de-epithelialized eyelid margin. This is run in a subcuticular fashion from upper to lower eyelid until exiting at the lateral canthus, where it is brought through skin and a bolster and each end is tied with a bulky knot. We use cut pieces of silicone tubing from a butterfly scalp vein catheter as my bolsters. The bolsters and Prolene suture can be removed after 3 weeks and a permanent adhesion will result.

The advantage of a permanent tarsorrhaphy performed in this fashion is that the tarsorrhaphy can be readily reversed by incising with Wescott scissors placed between the opposed eyelid margins. The bare tarsal margin will readily reepithelialize. If initial deepithelialization was carried out without excising the body of the tarsal plate, trichiasis should not be a problem (Figure 16-3).

Pillar Tarsorrhaphy

If it is important to examine the underlying ocular surface after permanent tarsorrhaphy, then a pillar tarsorrhaphy is useful. This is a more involved surgical procedure, in that it requires the development of medial and lateral tarsoconjunctival pillars from the upper eyelid that are sutured into corresponding medial and lateral recipient sites in the inferior fornix. The development of the upper eyelid tars-conjunctival pillars is similar to the technique used in development of a Hughes flap used in lower eyelid reconstruction (Figure 16-4). Two comparable pillars of proximal tarsal plate and a conjunctival-Müller's muscle pedicle each 4 to 5 mm in width are developed from the medial and lateral upper eyelid. These are advanced and sutured into medial and lateral recipient sites just proximal to the inferior border of the lower eyelid tarsal plate. The pedicles pull the upper eyelid margin down so that it opposes the lower eyelid margin. However, the pull of the tarsoconjunctival pedicle can be overcome with superior traction to allow the upper eyelid to be distracted upward and allow visualization of the underlying cornea. The pillars can be severed in the same fashion that a Hughes flap is taken down when corneal protection is no longer needed.

Tarsorrhaphy is an essential procedure in the management of numerous processes that may threaten the anterior segment of the eye. Although temporary procedures are often called for, slight modification of these will allow permanent (but reversible) closure when necessary.

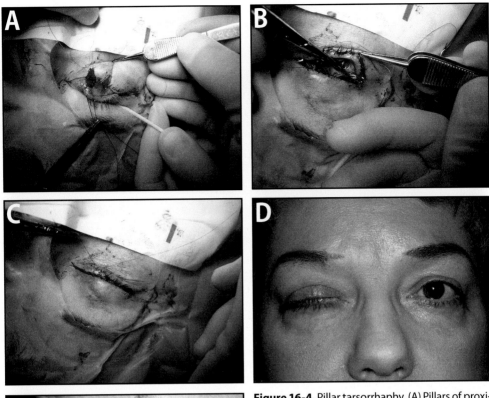

Figure 16-4. Pillar tarsorrhaphy. (A) Pillars of proximal tarsus and the attached conjunctivo-Müllers pedicle are developed from the proximal tarsus in the medial and lateral upper eyelid, spaced about 1 cm apart. (B) Two corresponding recipient beds are dissected in the palpebral conjunctiva of the lower eyelid just proximal to the inferior border of the lower eyelid tarsal plate. (C) The pedicles are sutured into the recipient sites with 5-0 Vicryl sutures, which exit through orbicularis and skin and are tied on the skin surface of the lower eyelid. (D) The eyelids are held in opposition by the pedicles. (E) The eyelid margin can be lifted to view the underlying anterior segment.

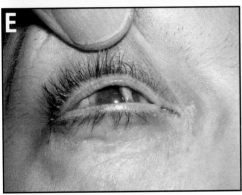

References

1. Banu CC, Cohen EJ, Rapuano CJ, et al. Tarsorrhaphy: clinical experience from a cornea practice. *Cornea.* 2001;20(8):787-791.
2. Schimek RA, Ballou GS. Eastman 910 monomer for plastic lid procedures. *Am J Ophthalmol.* 1966;62:953-955.
3. Kitchens J, Kinder J, Oetting T. The drawstring temporary tarsorrhaphy technique. *Arch Ophthalmol.* 2002;120:187-190.

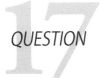

WHAT COMMERCIALLY AVAILABLE MATERIALS CAN BE USED AS TISSUE SUBSTITUTES IN EYELID RECONSTRUCTION?

Michael K. Yoon, MD and
N. Grace Lee, MD

I'm not very comfortable with eyelid reconstruction. In particular, I have trouble with anterior lamellar grafting and posterior lamellar spacers. What materials work best? How do the different options compare?

There are increasing numbers of commercially available grafts that can serve as posterior lamellar eyelid spacers or reconstructive grafts when autologous options are not possible. Allografts, which are derived from donor human tissue, include Tutoplast sclera (IOP Ophthalmics), AlloDerm (LifeCell), and DermaMatrix (Synthes). Enduragen (Tissue Science Laboratories) and tarSys (IOP Ophthalmics) are examples of xenografts (ie, nonhuman) of porcine origin that are also commercially available. Additionally, there is a synthetic, alloplastic Medpor graft (Stryker) that can be used to repair eyelid retraction. All tissue-derived materials have the benefit of commercial availability, which eliminates the need for a donor site and can decrease operative time. The risks of such materials include variable and unpredictable resorption, the risk for infection transmission, and the cost of the processed product. The selection of each graft type should be tailored to the individual patient.

Eyelid reconstruction can be categorized into 2 general types of surgery. The first is replacement of lost tissue following tumor excision (eg, after Mohs micrographic surgery) or other forms of trauma. The second is restoration of the normal eyelid position such as repair of eyelid retraction as a result of cosmetic blepharoplasty, surgical scarring, thyroid eye disease, or other conditions. To determine how the eyelids should be repaired, both the anterior and posterior lamellae of the eyelids must be considered.

The anterior lamella, consisting of the skin and orbicularis oculi muscle, can be directly closed or replaced by techniques such as advancement flaps, rotational flaps, skin grafts, or pedicle grafts. Deficiencies in this layer are not replaced with commercially available materials. Reconstruction of the posterior lamella, consisting of the tarsus and conjunctiva, has more limited options. These include direct closure, vascularized tarsoconjunctival flaps (eg, Hughes flaps), and replacement with autologous grafts or commercially available graft materials.

Kersten RC, McCulley TJ, eds. *Curbside Consultation in Oculoplastics:*
49 Clinical Questions, Second Edition (pp 89-92).
© 2016 Taylor & Francis Group.

Most surgeons will prefer to use direct tissue approximation or local flaps as a first line for closure of eyelid defects because this replaces lost tissue with similar tissue and can help maximize the likelihood of an excellent functional and cosmetic outcome. However, when this is precluded by extensive tissue loss, replacement flaps or grafts are needed. It is important to note the differences in the placement of tissue for eyelid reconstruction vs repair of eyelid retraction. In the former, the deficient tarsus is completely replaced by graft material, allowing the graft to come in contact with the cornea. In the latter, the existing tarsal plate is left in place, and additional material is placed between the proximal tarsal edge and the fornix conjunctiva as a spacer. In either setting, but especially with eyelid reconstruction, there is a risk for corneal abrasion when using these materials.

Ideal properties for grafts are biological compatibility, availability in abundance, an appropriate balance of rigidity and pliability, zero risk for infection transmission, and minimal and/or predictable resorption rates. Many surgeons prefer autologous tissues because they are often reliable, have no risk for infection transmission, and there is no immunologic risk. Commonly used autologous tissues include tarsus,[1] hard palate mucosa,[2] dermis,[3] and auricular cartilage.[4] However, the morbidity and potentially increased operative time when harvesting tissue may make this less desirable. Commercially available posterior lamellar tissue substitutes eliminate these limitations, although there is added cost, potential for significant resorption, and risk for disease transmission. Depending on the situation, commercially available tissue substitutes may best suit the patient. The materials for posterior lamellar replacement come in 3 general forms: allografts, xenografts, and alloplastic materials.

Allografts are materials that are derived from donor human tissue. These products have been processed by the manufacturer to prevent transmission of viruses and prions, as well as to remove immunogenic content. Although a theoretical risk for disease transmission still remains, this is considered to be unlikely.

Banked sclera or Tutoplast sclera is processed human cadaveric sclera consisting of decellularized collagen. This material is one of the earliest used donor tissues in ophthalmology and has been used for various purposes ranging from glaucoma surgery to anophthalmic socket repair. In the eyelid, it has been most frequently used to increase the vertical height of the eyelid. This material requires no preparation after opening the packaging. After placing the material onto the sterile field, it can be shaped to the desired size then sutured into place. The surface is smooth, preventing the need to bury it under conjunctiva or to place a bandage contact lens.[5] Investigations of this material have demonstrated significant resorption of the sclera, limiting the long-term effectiveness of the surgery.[6,7] Other authors have suggested that its thin, supple nature lacks adequate rigidity necessary for posterior lamellar support.[8] Thus, its use in eyelid retraction repair or reconstruction is rare.

Another allograft is a matrix of human cadaver dermis that has been processed to remove cells while a freeze-drying process removes moisture within the tissue. The structure of the remaining collagen matrix is left intact to allow ingrowth of the host vasculature and fibrosis. There are 2 products available: AlloDerm and DermaMatrix. These products have been used for repair or replacement of damaged or inadequate integumental tissue throughout the body. Uses in the eyelid are to replace deficient tarsus. Differences between the two products are that AlloDerm requires refrigerated storage, has a 2-year shelf life, and requires 10 to 40 minutes of rehydration prior to use. DermaMatrix can be stored without refrigeration for up to 3 years and requires 20 minutes of rehydration. There can be significant contraction of dermal matrix after implantation making its long-term effect on eyelid height unpredictable,[9] although no studies have compared these 2 materials. The graft should be properly oriented with the epidermal side facing the globe and the deep surface facing the orbital septum or orbicularis oculi muscle. The surface of these dermal matrices is not smooth until conjunctival coverage is complete, which may take up to 2 weeks.[10] When used in the upper eyelid especially, covering the posterior surface with conjunctiva or placing a bandage contact lens should be strongly considered.

Xenografts are materials that are derived from other species. One of the more commonly used materials in the eyelid is porcine collagen dermal matrix (Enduragen). It has similarities in the properties of allogenic dermal matrix, although some authors believe it is more durable and more consistent in thickness.[11] The material comes in thicknesses of 0.5 and 1.0 mm, with the thicker version used in the lower eyelid.[11] No rehydration or special preparation of the Enduragen is necessary prior to use. There has been no comparison of porcine to human dermal matrix, although Enduragen was observed to have little resorption in a single case where reoperation occurred after 6 months.[12] Similar to the allograft dermal matrices, Enduragen should be covered by conjunctiva or a bandage contact lens placed when used in the upper eyelid.

A newer material, tarSys, has been bioengineered from porcine small intestinal submucosa with specialized processing. It consists of 8 or 12 layers of decellularized membrane containing collagen types I, III, and VI. Unlike other materials, this is specifically designed for use in the eyelid. Prior to use intraoperatively, the tarSys graft must be rehydrated in sterile solution (with or without additional antibiotic) for at least 20 minutes. Some authors recommend using a 4-to-1 ratio of tarSys height to desired eyelid change.[8] The graft can then be placed into the bed and sutured into place. There is no need to orient this material. There is only a case report and a single retrospective, noncomparative series that demonstrated safety and efficacy for lower eyelid retraction.[8,13] Unpublished experiences have claimed success in eyelid reconstruction after tumor removal and trauma.[14] Criticisms of the material include observations that the material can melt during periods of resorption and produce white mucoid discharge.[8] Finally, as a porcine xenograft, the risk for transmitting infectious agents or allergic inflammation exist.

One alloplastic material available for eyelid surgery is the Medpor lower eyelid spacer. This is a porous polyethylene sheet that is used for repair of lower eyelid retraction due to scarring of the orbital septum or posterior lamella, particularly following cosmetic lower blepharoplasty. This rigid biomaterial mechanically elevates the lower eyelid while its pores allow vascular ingrowth and integration to maintain it in place.[15] This rigid and rough sheet must be implanted with posterior coverage by conjunctiva to prevent abrasion of the ocular surface. Its stiffness allows for effective elevation of the retracted lower eyelids, but is not intended for reconstruction of the posterior lamella. However, frequent erosion and exposure of the porous polyethylene has limited its popularity.[16]

The number of commercially available materials available to the surgeon for eyelid reconstruction continues to increase and each has its own benefits and drawbacks. The choice of graft type should be determined based on its applicability to the individual patient, the most important tissue characteristics needed for reconstruction, and familiarity with the material and technique.

References

1. Stephenson CM, Brown BZ. The use of tarsus as a free autogenous graft in eyelid surgery. *Ophthal Plast Reconstr Surg.* 1985;1:43-50.
2. Kersten RC, Kulwin DR, Levartovsky S, Tiradellis H, Tse DT. Management of lower-lid retraction with hard palate mucosa grafting. *Arch Ophthalmol.* 1990;108:1339-1343.
3. Yoon MK, McCulley TJ. Autologous dermal grafts as posterior lamellar spacers in the management of lower eyelid retraction. *Ophthal Plast Reconstr Surg.* 2014;30(1):64-68.
4. Baylis HI, Perman KI, Fett DR, et al. Autogenous auricular cartilage grafting for lower eyelid retraction. *Ophthal Plast Reconstr Surg.* 1985;1:23-27.
5. Flanagan JC. Retraction of the eyelids secondary to thyroid ophthalmopathy—its surgical correction with sclera and the fate of the graft. *Trans Am Ophth Soc.* 1980;89:657-685.
6. Doxanas MT, Dryden RM. The use of sclera in the treatment of dysthyroid eyelid retraction. *Ophthalmology.* 1981;88(9):887-894.
7. Mourits MP, Koorneef L. Lid lengthening by sclera interposition for eyelid retraction in Graves' ophthalmopathy. *Br J Ophthalmol.* 1991;75(6):344-347.

8. Liao SL, Wei YS. Correction of lower lid retraction using tarSys bioengineered grafts for Graves' ophthalmopathy. *Am J Ophthalmol*. 2013;156:387-392.
9. Sullivan SA, Dailey RA. Graft contraction: a comparison of acellular dermis versus hard palate mucosa in lower eyelid surgery. *Ophthal Plast Reconstr Surg*. 2003;19(1):14-24.
10. Taban M, Douglas R, Li T, et al. Efficacy of "thick" acellular human dermis (AlloDerm) for lower eyelid reconstruction. *Arch Facial Plast Surg*. 2005;7:38-44.
11. Symbas J, McCord C, Nahai F. Acellular dermal matrix in eyelid surgery. *Aesthet Surg J*. 2011;31:101S-107S.
12. McCord C, Nahai FR, Codner MA, et al. Use of porcine acellular dermal matrix (Enduragen) grafts in eyelids: a review of 69 patients and 129 eyelids. *Plast Reconstr Surg*. 2008;122:1206-1213.
13. Borrelli M, Unterlauft J, Kleinsasser N, Geerling G. Decellularized porcine derived membrane (tarSys) for correction of lower eyelid retraction. *Orbit*. 2012;31(3):187-189.
14. Aakalu VK, Elderkin S, Weiss RA. Effective use of tarSys bioengineered eyelid prostheses for eyelid reconstruction. In: The Association for Research in Vision and Ophthalmology Annual Meeting; May 3-7, 2009; Fort Lauderdale, Florida. Abstract 5059.
15. Wong JF, Soparkar CN, Patrinely JR. Correction of lower eyelid retraction with high density porous polyethylene: the Medpor lower eyelid spacer. *Orbit*. 2001;20(3):217-225.
16. Tan J, Olver J, Wright M, et al. The use of porous polyethylene (Medpor) lower eyelid spacers in lid heightening and stabilisation. *Br J Ophthalmol*. 2004;88:1197-2000.

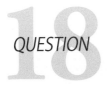

WHEN DO YOU WORRY THAT AN EYELID GROWTH IS MALIGNANT?

Robert Alan Goldberg, MD

I often notice small growths on my patients' eyelids. When should I be concerned? Do you have any tips for identifying malignancy?

Screening for eyelid skin cancer should be a routine component of the eye exam, and early identification of a skin cancer can make an enormous impact on the lives of our patients. The difference between early and late detection can mean acceptable cosmetic results rather than a disfiguring outcome, saving the eye instead of losing it, or even saving the patient's life instead of death from metastatic or invasive cancer.

The problem is that early cancers can sometimes look like benign inflammatory or reactive processes such as a chalazion, blepharitis, nevus (mole), or dermatitis. As ophthalmologists, we can take advantage of the biomicroscope. The slit-lamp gives a magnified stereo view that can reveal fantastic details about the anatomy of a skin lesion, and can often allow accurate diagnosis of the skin cancer of the eyelids at a very early stage.

What are the features of skin cancer that can be observed clinically? The answer lies in understanding the biology of cancer. Microscopically, cancer cells grow and replace normal tissue. That replacement of tissue results in destruction of normal architecture. The architecture of the eyelid margin is beautifully complex, and destruction of that architecture can be recognized readily by the trained eye.

When screening for architectural changes, there are several common clues that should be sought.

Kersten RC, McCulley TJ, eds. *Curbside Consultation in Oculoplastics: 49 Clinical Questions, Second Edition* (pp 93-95).
© 2016 Taylor & Francis Group.

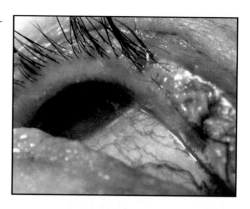

Figure 18-1. Sebaceous carcinoma with loss of meibomian gland architecture in the lateral upper eyelid.

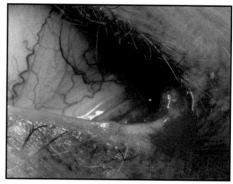

Figure 18-2. Basal cell carcinoma lower eyelid with loss of the smooth, sharp mucocutaneous junction.

Loss of Eyelashes

Eyelashes can fall out temporarily in response to inflammation such as blepharitis. However, complete and persistent eyelash loss—especially in one focal area—should raise the suspicion of neoplasia.

Loss of Meibomian Gland Architecture

There is no benign process that causes loss of meibomian gland architecture. The regular, repeating architecture of the individual meibomian glands—at the eyelid margin as well as the posterior tarsal surface—can be easily visualized via the slit-lamp. A process that results in loss of meibomian gland architecture (replaced by monotonous undifferentiated tissue) is highly suspicious for neoplasia (Figure 18-1).

Loss of the "Windshield Wiper"

The sharp line of the mucocutaneous junction forms the windshield wiper that spreads the tear film on the cornea. This sharp line can be identified by its smooth reflection. Loss of the smooth, sharp mucocutaneous junction is a clinical feature that should raise suspicion of a neoplastic process that may be invading this normal epithelial transition (Figure 18-2).

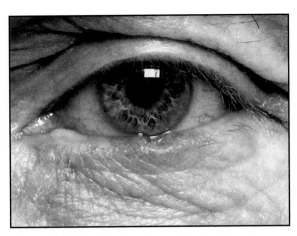

Figure 18-3. Classic rodent ulcer of basal cell carcinoma.

Ulcerated Skin or Chronic Scabbing

The classic basal cell carcinoma of the eyelid margin has a fairly white, shiny, smooth elevation with fine blood vessels seen under the slit-lamp and a central ulcer that has a wet appearance because of the lack of epithelium. The region replaces normal tissue so the architecture is destroyed. When the classic appearance of a rodent ulcer is present, we can make the diagnosis of basal cell carcinoma with high certainty (Figure 18-3). Other skin cancers such as squamous carcinoma also cause loss of the epithelium, often with chronic crusting or bleeding.

Unilateral Severe Blepharitis

Sebaceous carcinoma is the most dangerous common eyelid cancer, and it can be the most difficult to diagnose. Instead of starting in the epithelium, it starts further back in the meibomian glands in the tarsal plate. It also tends to spread through the tissues quickly, without making a large, elevated bump. Therefore, it can present as a diffuse red eyelid and be confused with blepharitis. Careful examination will usually reveal evidence of destructive changes such as loss of meibomian orifices or absence of eyelashes. Persistent blepharitis on one side or in a focal area of an eyelid should raise suspicion for sebaceous carcinoma and lead to a careful analysis for destruction of eyelid margin architecture.

By understanding how microscopic tissue changes are reflected in what we visualize through the slit-lamp, and by tuning in to the microscopic architecture of the eyelid margin and typical patterns of architectural destruction, many eyelid malignancies can be identified early, biopsied, and appropriately treated. Early detection and treatment can be vision sparing or sometimes even life sparing.

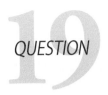

WHEN SHOULD MOHS SURGERY BE EMPLOYED?

Isaac M. Neuhaus, MD

What is Mohs surgery? How does it compare to just using frozen sections? When should Mohs excision be used in the management of eyelid tumors? Are there any types of tumors that should not be excised with Mohs surgery?

Mohs micrographic surgery, named after its developer Dr. Frederic Mohs, is the preferred method to excise many skin malignancies. The main advantage to Mohs surgery is preservation of uninvolved tissue and evaluation of the entire surgical margins. A surgeon's approach to skin cancer excision is balanced by 2 conflicting tenets. On the one hand, wide excision is required to ensure complete removal of the neoplasm. Competing with this is the need to spare as much normal tissue adjacent to the tumor as possible to facilitate reconstruction to reduce the impact on both cosmesis and function. Mohs micrographic surgery is a surgical technique that allows for optimal balance between margin control and tissue conservation. In this technique, the physician acts as both the surgeon and pathologist to obtain the highest cure rate possible. In almost all cases, Mohs surgery is performed under local anesthesia in an outpatient setting, thus adding to the safety of the surgery.

Traditional pathologic evaluation of excised tissue employs a bread-loaf technique, whether with permanent formalin-fixed slides or frozen tissue examination at the time of surgery. Vertical cut step sections are taken throughout the specimen, but only allow for examination of less than 0.1% of the surgical margin. As a result, the tumor may extend to the margin in the areas between the sections, resulting in a possibility of recurrence due to inadequate excision. Surgeons can compensate for this pathologic limitation by taking a more substantial surgical margin to ensure adequate extirpation of the tumor, albeit with a greater impact on reconstruction options due to the larger size of the resulting defect. This is particularly detrimental when dealing with the eyelids, where a large number of critical structures are within millimeters of each other.

Kersten RC, McCulley TJ, eds. *Curbside Consultation in Oculoplastics:*
49 Clinical Questions, Second Edition (pp 97-100).
© 2016 Taylor & Francis Group.

Figure 19-1. (A) This 75-year-old woman has a new diagnosis of basal cell carcinoma on the lower lid. (B) The tumor was found to extend beyond the grossly abnormal borders; note the relatively large size of the defect.

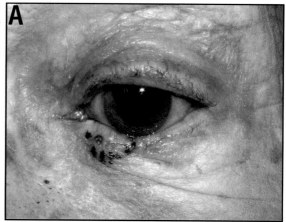

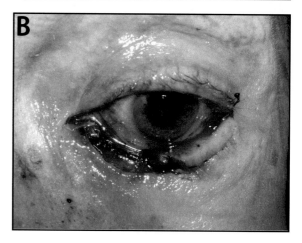

In contrast to traditional excision and pathologic evaluation, Mohs micrographic surgery uses horizontal sections to evaluate 100% of the surgical margin. The tissue is excised with an angled bevel, which can then be placed flat on the frozen sections. A useful analogy is to think of the excised specimen as an orange peel that is laid flat on the slide. By carefully examining the entire surgical margin in this manner, one can identify any residual tumor and map it to a precise anatomic location. This is in contrast to traditional frozen sections, which use the same bread loaf described previously and can only identify a positive margin if it is in the small portion of surgical margin examined. Subsequent Mohs stages are directed only to the areas of positive tumor, with the remaining clear sections undisturbed. The process is repeated until the entire tumor is removed, with the patient waiting between stages while the slides are made and examined. In many cases, the tumor ends up being significantly larger than might be expected based on the preoperative size (Figure 19-1). By using careful microscopic control of surgical margins, the Mohs surgeon can obtain an improved clearance rate compared to standard excision, while minimizing the amount of normal tissue removed.

Following clearance of the tumor, the wound can be immediately reconstructed, allowed to heal by second intention, or have delayed reconstruction. In most cases, the Mohs surgeon performs the reconstruction, but referral to another physician (an oculoplastic surgeon in this case) can be considered. When coordinating with an oculoplastic surgeon, the reconstruction is usually performed within 24 hours, although a longer delay is acceptable if there is a logistical challenge. The advantage for the reconstructing surgeon would be the assurance that the tumor is removed, thus giving the surgeon a greater degree of freedom when considering repair options.

Mohs surgery is used for a variety of tumors, including basal cell carcinoma, squamous cell carcinoma, keratoacanthoma, Merkel cell carcinoma, dermatofibrosarcoma protuberans, atypical fibroxanthoma, microcystic adnexal carcinoma, sebaceous carcinoma, and extramammary Paget's disease. Cure rates vary depending on the specific tumor being treated. Primary basal cell carcinoma treated with Mohs surgery has a 99% 5-year cure rate (vs 90% for standard treatments). Recurrent basal cell carcinoma treated with Mohs surgery has a 5-year cure rate of 94% (vs 80% for standard treatments). Similar results can be obtained for different tumors.

Indications for Mohs surgery also include recurrent or incompletely excised tumors, tumors with aggressive histologic growth patterns (eg, infiltrative, micronodular, perivascular, perineural), or tumors with indistinct clinical margins. In addition to specific tumor characteristics, tumors in high-risk anatomic areas, where recurrence or extensive excision may result in either cosmetic or functional deficits, are candidates for Mohs surgery. Patients with a high risk for multiple tumors (eg, those that are immunosuppressed, have a history of solid organ transplant, basal cell nevus syndrome, or xeroderma pigmentosum) can be treated with Mohs surgery.

Any tumor with a discontiguous growth pattern is not a candidate for Mohs surgery, given the possibility that tumor may be present beyond a clear margin. In addition, the tumor must be visible on frozen sections. Thus, if the tumor subtype has unreliable histologic features on frozen sections, Mohs surgery should not be used. The most common tumor falling into this category is melanoma. This is currently an area of debate, with some advocating for the use of Mohs surgery and others preferring that the melanoma be excised and evaluated with traditional permanent sections. Also worth noting, Mohs surgery is primarily used to evaluate margins; if there is still a question of the diagnosis, a traditional pathologic exam is indicated.

Summary

Mohs surgery is the preferred method for excising many malignancies of the eyelid. Mohs surgery allows for preservation of most normal tissue without compromising judicious excision. It is common practice for Mohs surgeons to work in conjunction with an oculoplastic surgeon, who performs the reconstruction of the eyelid.

Suggested Readings

Harvey DT, Taylor RS, Itani KM, Loewinger RJ. Mohs micrographic surgery of the eyelid: an overview of anatomy, pathophysiology, and reconstruction options. *Dermatol Surg.* 2013;39(5):673-697.

Lindgren G, Lindblom B, Bratel AT, Mölne L, Larkö O. Mohs' micrographic surgery for basal cell carcinomas on the eyelids and medial canthal area. I. Characteristics of the tumours and details of the procedure. *Acta Ophthalmol Scand.* 2000;78(4):425-429.

Lindgren G, Lindblom B, Larkö O. Mohs' micrographic surgery for basal cell carcinomas on the eyelids and medial canthal area. II. Reconstruction and follow-up. *Acta Ophthalmol Scand.* 2000;78(4):430-436.

Malhotra R, Huilgol SC, Huynh NT, Selva D. The Australian Mohs database: periocular squamous cell carcinoma. *Ophthalmology.* 2004;111(4):617-623.

Malhotra R, Huilgol SC, Huynh NT, Selva D. The Australian Mohs database, part I: periocular basal cell carcinoma experience over 7 years. *Ophthalmology.* 2004;111(4):624-630.

Malhotra R, Huilgol SC, Huynh NT, Selva D. The Australian Mohs database, part II: periocular basal cell carcinoma outcome at 5-year follow-up. *Ophthalmology.* 2004;111(4):631-636.

Mohs FE. Micrographic surgery for the microscopically controlled excision of eyelid cancers. *Arch Ophthalmol.* 1986;104(6):901-909.

Monheit GD, Callahan MA, Callahan A. Mohs micrographic surgery for periorbital skin cancer. *Dermatol Clin.* 1989;7(4):677-697.

Slutsky JB, Jones EC. Periocular cutaneous malignancies: a review of the literature. *Dermatol Surg.* 2012;38(4):552-569.

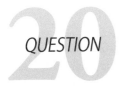

SHOULD PERIOCULAR CAPILLARY HEMANGIOMAS BE TREATED WITH CORTICOSTEROIDS, BETA-BLOCKERS, OR SURGERY?

Roxana Rivera, MD

I recently heard that there are new treatments for capillary hemangiomas. Have you tried beta-blockers? Are they safer than steroid injections?

Infantile hemangioma (IH) is the most common vascular tumor of infancy. It occurs more frequently in females (2:1 ratio), Whites, premature births, and products of multiple gestations.[1] IHs are not present at birth, but develop in the first few weeks of life. They vary widely in appearance, size, and depth of cutaneous involvement. IH is often subclassified as superficial, deep, or mixed; or localized/focal, segmental, or indeterminate. IHs exhibit a proliferative phase with rapid growth starting at 2 to 3 weeks of life until 5 to 9 months of age, followed by a plateau phase from 9 to 12 months of age, and then variably start to involute around 12 months up until 5 to 10 years of age.[2]

Although benign, IHs have a high rate of complications including ulceration, bleeding, infection, visual obstruction, airway obstruction, and residual scarring and disfigurement.[1] Pharmacologic or surgical treatment is reserved for such complicated IHs. Periocular IHs pose the risk for causing amblyopia by deprivation, astigmatism, or strabismus that can lead to severe and life-long visual impairment. Obstruction of the visual axis leads to severe amblyopia. For periocular IHs interfering with visual development, early treatment is critical.

Corticosteroids

Corticosteroids have been the mainstay of medical treatment for IHs since their incidental discovery in the 1960s. Intralesional injection of corticosteroids has been the mainstay therapy for vision-threatening periocular IHs due to its efficacy, convenience, and rare systemic side effects.[3,4] Janmohamed et al[5] reported a series of 34 patients with periocular IH treated with intralesional

Kersten RC, McCulley TJ, eds. *Curbside Consultation in Oculoplastics: 49 Clinical Questions, Second Edition* (pp 101-104).
© 2016 Taylor & Francis Group.

corticosteroids. Ninety-one percent of patients showed regression at 12 months. Five patients needed a second injection. There were no reported complications.

However, intralesional injection of corticosteroids in the head and neck region can result in ocular embolization with permanent loss of vision.[6,7] Two necessary conditions for ocular embolization are (1) intravascular injection with retrograde flow caused by high-injection pressures exceeding the mean systemic arterial pressure, and (2) a sufficient volume of intravascular corticosteroid injected at such high pressures.[8] Some investigators advocate the use of a large-capacity syringe and a small-bore cannula to decrease the injection pressure.[9] I use a 10-cc syringe with a 27-gauge needle.

The corticosteroid combination most frequently used is a 50:50 mixture of triamcinolone acetonide (40 mg/mL Kenalog-40; Bristol-Myers Squibb) and a mixture of betamethasone acetate and betamethasone sodium phosphate (6 mg/mL Celestone Soluspan; Schering Co). We recommend limiting the volume injected to less than 1.5 cc per lesion.

Samimi et al[9] reported a series of 50 patients with amblyogenic eyelid capillary hemangiomas treated with intralesional corticosteroid injection. They described an injection technique that minimizes the risk for central retinal artery occlusion. They advocate placing the needle perpendicular to the arterial vessels in the vicinity of the tumor or parallel to the regional arterial vessels and pointed in the direction of the vessels' forward flow to avoid arterial cannulation. An assistant applies digital compression on the supraorbital vascular bundle and the corticosteroid is injected slowly while withdrawing the needle from the lesion core. In their series, all 50 patients demonstrated a reduction in tumor size; 4 lesions required a second injection. None of the patients developed a retinal vascular occlusion. Indirect ophthalmoscopy during or after intralesional injection of corticosteroids in the periorbital area is highly recommended.

Beta-Blockers

Since Léauté-Labrèze et al[10] in 2008 fortuitously discovered the efficacy of beta-blockers for the treatment of IH, multiple reports and studies have substantiated the usefulness of this drug in periocular IH. Most of these publications are not prospective, randomized, or controlled.

Spiteri-Cornish and Reddy[11] performed a systematic review of the literature published on the use of propranolol in the management of periocular capillary hemangiomas. They found 19 articles with a total of 100 cases (1 week to 18 months of age) of oral propranolol use in periorbital or orbital capillary hemangiomas. Of the 85 cases that had details of previous treatment, propranolol was used as first-line treatment in 50 (58.8%). The most common dose used was 2 mg/kg per day. Adverse events were documented in 26 of the 100 cases. Most of the adverse effects were minor. However, in 3 cases (3%), propranolol was discontinued due to bronchospasm (n = 1), symptomatic hypoglycemia (n = 1), and hypotension (n = 1). Improvement or complete resolution of the lesions occurred in 96% of cases. Recurrence was noted in 15% of cases.

The literature published since 2008 on the use of propranolol in IH shows significant divergence of opinion regarding indications for use, dosing, and safety monitoring. To address some of these issues, a consensus conference was held in December 2011 with 28 participants from 12 institutions, representing 5 specialties.[12] Their recommendations include starting propranolol at 1 mg/kg per day divided 3 times daily with a target dose of 1 to 3 mg/kg/day. They recommend that the 20 mg/5mL preparation of propranolol be used. Inpatient hospitalization for initiation of propranolol is suggested for infants <8 weeks of gestationally corrected age or with comorbid conditions. Patient heart rate and blood pressure should be measured at baseline and at 1 and 2 hours after receiving the initial dose, and after significant dose increase (>0.5 mg/kg per day). Propranolol should be discontinued during intercurrent illness or restricted oral intake to prevent hypoglycemia.[12]

A multidisciplinary approach is ideal in the management of IH with propranolol. Every patient should be screened for risks associated with propranolol use and a cardiovascular and pulmonary history and examination should be performed by a care provider with experience in evaluating infants and children.

To date, there are no published randomized controlled trials on the efficacy and safety of propranolol in the treatment of periocular IH. International multicenter studies on the use of propranolol in IH are currently underway, including an active phase II/III Investigational New Drug application (Clinicaltrials.gov NCT01056341).

Surgery

Although corticosteroids and propranolol are highly efficacious in the treatment of IHs, some lesions do not respond to these medications. The risk factors for nonresponse include focalized IH, central upper and lower face localization and IH with both superficial and deep components.[13]

For periocular hemangiomas that are causing significant amblyopia, surgery may be the most effective, timely, and safe modality to achieve equal visual development.[14]

The advantages of surgical excision include immediate resolution of amblyogenic factors (deprivation, astigmatism) and disfigurement. This must be balanced against the increased risk for bleeding in small infants with limited blood volume. When completed early, surgical excision provides definitive therapy, preventing local recurrence.

Summary

Given the high variability in the presentation of periocular IH, the treatment plan should be individualized, considering variables such as the location of the hemangioma, rate of growth, potential for inducing amblyopia, as well as the overall health of the patient and individual risk factors for each treatment alternative.

References

1. Haggstrom AN, Drolet BA, Baselga E, et al. Prospective study of infantile hemangiomas: clinical characteristics predicting complications and treatment. *Pediatrics*. 2006;118(3):882-887.
2. Chang LC, Haggstrom AN, Drolet BA. Hemangioma Investigator Group. Growth characteristics of infantile hemangiomas: implications for management. *Pediatrics*. 2008;122(2):360-367.
3. Kushner BJ. The treatment of periorbital infantile hemangioma with intralesional corticosteroid. *Plast Reconstr Surg*. 1985;76:517-526.
4. Weiss AH, Kelly JP. Reappraisal of astigmatism induced by periocular capillary hemangioma and treatment with intralesional corticosteroid injection. *Ophthalmology*. 2008;115(2):390-397.
5. Janmohamed SR, Madern GC, Nieuwenhuis K, de Laat PC, Oranje AP. Evaluation of intralesional corticosteroids in the treatment of periocular hemangioma of infancy: still an alternative besides propranolol. *Pediatr Surg Int*. 2012;28(4):393-398.
6. Shorr N, Seiff SR. Central retinal artery occlusion associated with periocular corticosteroid injection for juvenile hemangioma. *Ophthalmic Surg*. 1986;17:229-231.
7. Ruttum MS, Abrams GH, Harris GH, Ellis MK. Bilateral retinal embolization associated with intralesional corticosteroid injection for capillary hemangioma of infancy. *J Pediatr Ophthalmol Strabismus*. 1993;30:4-7.
8. Egbert JE, Saurav P, Engel WK, Summers CG. High injection pressure during intralesional injection of corticosteroids into capillary hemangiomas. *Arch Ophthalmol*. 2001;119:677-683.
9. Samimi DB, Alabiad CR, Tse DT. An anatomically based approach to intralesional corticosteroid injection for eyelid capillary hemangiomas. *Ophthalmic Surg Lasers Imaging*. 2012;43:190-195.

10. Léauté-Labrèze C, Dumas de la Roque E, Hubiche T, Boralevi F, Thambo JB, Taïeb A. Propranolol for severe he-mangiomas of infancy. *N Engl J Med*. 2008;358(24):2649-2651.
11. Spiteri-Cornish K, Reddy AR. The use of propranolol in the management of periocular capillary hemangioma: a systematic review. *Eye (Lond)*. 2011;25(10):1277-1283.
12. Drolet BA, Frommelt PC, Chamlin SL, et al. Initiation and use of propranolol for infantile hemangioma: report of a consensus conference. *Pediatrics*. 2013;131(1):128-140.
13. Huoh KC, Rosbe KW. Infantile hemangiomas of the head and neck. *Pediatr Clin North Am*. 2013;60(4): 937-949.
14. Mawn LA. Infantile hemangioma: treatment with surgery or steroids. *Am Orthopt J*. 2013;63:6-13.

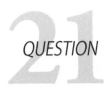

WHEN DOES AN EYELID LESION NEED TO BE BIOPSIED?

Richard Collin, MA, FRCS, FRCOphth, DO and
Michèle Beaconsfield, DO, FRCS, FRCOphth, FEBO

Do benign-appearing papillomas need to be biopsied? If a lesion looks benign, do I still need to send it to pathology? In what do I send the specimen: formalin, saline, or without solution all together? How should I do an eyelid biopsy? When is a full-thickness biopsy necessary? What do you do with an unsuspected skin lesion that proves to be malignant after excision in the office?

Eyelid lesions are notoriously difficult to diagnose accurately on the history and appearance alone (Figures 21-1 and 21-2). In one study by Kersten et al, roughly 2% of benign-appearing lesions turned out to be histologically malignant.[1] More importantly, there was no growth pattern that was uniformly seen in benign lesions. Therefore, we recommend biopsy and histological examination of any acquired and/or changing eyelid lesion. Whatever the appearance of the lesion, it does need to be sent for histology.

There are several malignant lesions that are infamous for their tendency to masquerade as benign lesions. Of course, the most notorious is a sebaceous or adenocarcinoma, which can resemble blepharitis, a chalazion, or sometimes a less aggressive basal cell carcinoma (BCC) (Figure 21-3). Squamous cell carcinomas (SCC) can appear like a benign papilloma, such as seborrheic keratosis. They may also present similarly to a keratoacanthoma (Figure 21-4). To be fair, there are those who consider keratoacanthomas to be a subgroup of SCC. Be particularly wary of melanotic lesions. Adults rarely acquire a nevus; therefore, no matter how benign in appearance, all acquired nevi in adults beyond the third decade should be biopsied (Figure 21-5).

Figure 21-6 illustrates the various ways to biopsy an eyelid lesion. An eyelid lesion biopsy can usually be carried out under local anesthetic. If the lesion is small, it can be removed with an excisional biopsy and the skin edges sutured, or the defect cauterized and left to granulate (Figure 21-7). If the lesion is larger, an incisional biopsy may be required. This classically involves taking a piece of the abnormal-looking lesion with an adjacent piece of normal-looking skin so that the

Kersten RC, McCulley TJ, eds. *Curbside Consultation in Oculoplastics:*
49 Clinical Questions, Second Edition (pp 105-108).

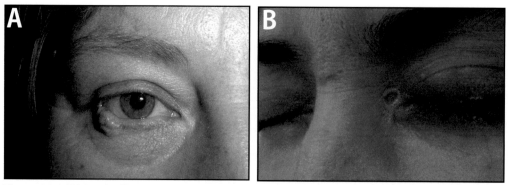

Figure 21-1. (A) Basal cell carcinomas usually present with elevated pearly borders and a central crater, (B) but can present with any number of less characteristic patterns.

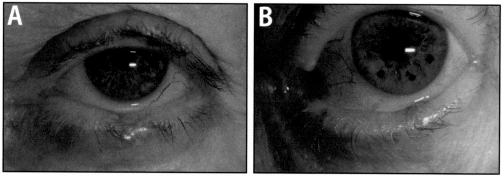

Figure 21-2. Two similarly appearing lesions: (A) a basal cell carcinoma and (B) an early chalazion.

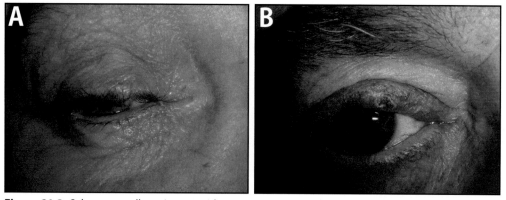

Figure 21-3. Sebaceous cell carcinoma with an appearance similar to (A) a chalazion, and (B) a basal cell carcinoma.

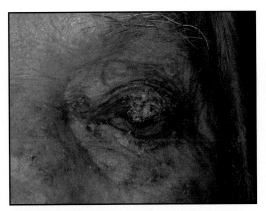

Figure 21-4. Squamous cell carcinoma with an appearance similar to a keratoacanthoma.

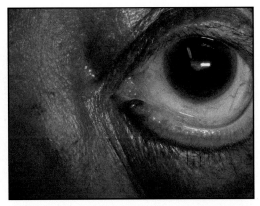

Figure 21-5. Malignant melanoma of the lower eyelid, which clinically resembles a benign nevus.

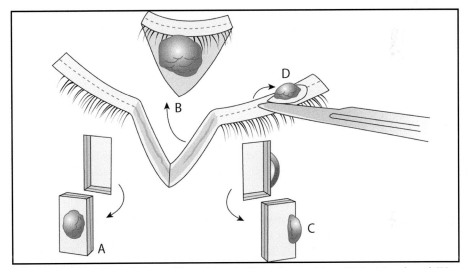

Figure 21-6. Biopsy technique: (A) excisional, (B) wedge excision, (C) incisional, and (D) a shave biopsy.

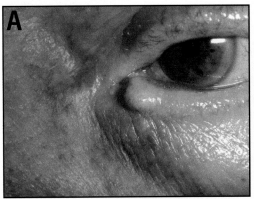
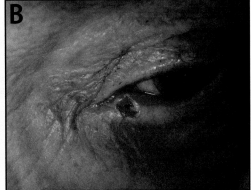

Figure 21-7. Following excision of small benign-appearing lesions, small wounds do not need to be closed and may be left to granulate.

junction between the two can be examined. The specimen should be removed as a small ellipse or as a "slice of cake." Any bleeding is stopped with cautery and the defect is allowed to heal by secondary intention. If the lesion is shallow and extends along the lid margin, it can be removed with a shave excision biopsy with cautery to the base. If it is a full-thickness "slice of cake" or pentagonal resection, the defect should be closed in layers.

There are a few unique circumstances. If the lesion is suspected of being a malignant melanoma, a punch biopsy should be done to assess the vertical depth of the lesion. A punch biopsy yields a full-thickness section of skin and even subcutaneous fat, if desired. This is very important in determining risk of metastases and ancillary treatment. A full-thickness biopsy is classically indicated when a sebaceous cell carcinoma is suspected, which is usually best achieved with a wedge resection. Alternately, a punch biopsy of the abnormal area of tarsal plate can be performed from the underside of the eyelid. This is important because these most often arise from the meibomian glands within the tarsus. The overlying skin may look indurated and inflamed but may not contain neoplastic cells.

Biopsy specimens should be sent routinely in formalin so that they can be processed and examined as a paraffin section. If a specific lesion such as a sebaceous cell carcinoma is suspected, the specimen may be better sent fresh (ie, wrapped in a saline-soaked gauze). Although formalin will not alter the ability to perform fat stains, routine processing of the specimen in alcohol will dissolve the fat, making the diagnosis of sebaceous carcinoma more difficult. Sending the tissue fresh precludes processing in alcohol. If it is necessary to send the tissue in formalin, the pathologist must be made aware that fat stains are being requested.

When biopsying a suspected malignancy, it is customary to perform an incisional biopsy, leaving some behind. This identifies the spot for further excision, ensuring clear margins. Occasionally, the situation arises when an excisional biopsy was performed on a benign-appearing lesion that turned out to be malignant. If well-healed, the exact location of the lesion may be difficult to determine. If the margins are clear, the patient can be followed up routinely. If the histology shows a relatively benign lesion that should not metastasize, such as a BCC, less than 50% of incompletely excised BCCs or SCCs recur and it is thus acceptable to consider observation provided the patient is aware of the need for continued prolonged observation. A deciding factor is location. If it occurred in the middle of the lower or upper eyelid, a recurrent lesion will be readily visible. Therefore, it is reasonable to offer the patient the choice of conservative management with observation and further excision only if a recurrence occurs. If the original site of the lesion was at the canthi, where a recurrence may not be easy to identify, we feel an attempt should be made to identify the original site of excision where a second biopsy can be taken. If there is no indication of the initial biopsy site, a map biopsy can be considered. Regardless of the decision, if no further tumor is identified, it is important to follow the patient closely for recurrence.

Summary

We recommend a biopsy for all acquired or changing eyelid lesions. Due to the difficulty in accurately making a diagnosis based on clinical features alone, all lesions should be sent for microscopic evaluation. No single biopsy technique can be used in all situations.

Reference

1. Kersten RC, Ewing-Chow D, Kulwin DR, Gallon M. Accuracy of clinical diagnosis of cutaneous eyelid lesions. *Ophthalmology.* 1997;104(3):479-484.

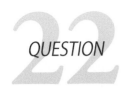
HOW SHOULD LENTIGO MALIGNA BE MANAGED?

Bishr Al Dabagh, MD; Linda C. Chang, MD;
Murray Cotter, MD, PhD; and Siegrid S. Yu, MD

What is lentigo maligna? Is there any difference between lentigo maligna and melanoma in situ? What is the malignant potential of lentigo maligna? If I suspect a lesion is lentigo maligna, how should it be assessed? Once confirmed, how do I manage it?

Lentigo maligna (LM) is a form of melanoma in situ (MIS) that occurs on chronically sun-damaged skin and is most frequently seen on the face in the seventh decade.[1] It often presents as an atypical, slow-growing, pigmented patch with some color variation and an irregular border (Figures 22-1 and 22-2). Delayed diagnosis is common, and clinical margins are often ill-defined. Recognition of LM is important because it can be a precursor to its invasive counterpart, lentigo maligna melanoma (LMM).[2]

LMM is 1 of 4 major subtypes of primary cutaneous melanoma. The estimated lifetime risk for LM progressing to LMM is not well defined, but has been estimated to be about 5% in one study.[2] More recent series have noted foci of invasion in as high as 16% of cases.[3] While the risk for progression is likely low, the prognosis for LMM is the same as that of any other melanoma of equivalent Breslow depth.

In the past, there has been some variation in the use of the term *lentigo maligna*. Some pathologists still refer to the reactive increase in atypical melanocytes induced by photodamage as LM, and distinguish this from melanoma in situ based on the extent and number of atypical melanocytes. In general, though, given the potential progression of LM to invasive LMM, most currently practicing dermatologists and dermatopathologists equate LM to melanoma in situ and will diagnose and treat lesions as such.[4] Further discussion on LM in this summary is in reference to it as one form of melanoma in situ.

During the physical examination, 2 useful tools can help the clinician decide whether the lesion warrants a biopsy. The first is epiluminescence microscopy, also known as dermoscopy.

Kersten RC, McCulley TJ, eds. *Curbside Consultation in Oculoplastics:*
49 Clinical Questions, Second Edition (pp 109-112).
© 2016 Taylor & Francis Group.

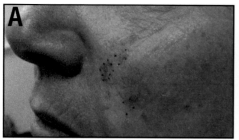
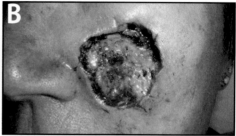

Figure 22-1. Lentigo maligna involving the left cheek. (A) Lentigo maligna can have significant subclinical extension. True margins may be difficult to appreciate preoperatively. (B) Postoperative photograph after clear margins were obtained.

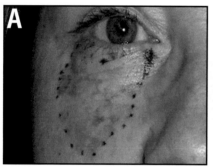
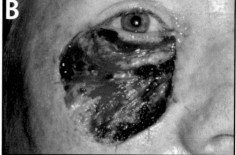

Figure 22-2. Periocular lentigo maligna. Standard surgical excision with 5- to 10-mm margins can be difficult in certain anatomic locations.

This instrument magnifies and illuminates the lesion and allows the clinician to look for findings associated with LM. Another useful tool is the Wood's lamp (ultraviolet lamp), which can highlight subtle hyperpigmentation and help better estimate the true borders of the pigmented lesion for diagnostic and therapeutic purposes. More recently, in vivo reflectance confocal microscopy has been used to delineate margins prior to treatment and has been found to be superior to dermoscopy.[5]

Lesions suspicious for LM should be biopsied. Ideally, an excisional biopsy of the entire lesion should be performed, as partial or incisional biopsies are subject to sampling error. If the suspicious lesion covers a large, cosmetically sensitive area where it would be difficult to start with an excisional biopsy, it is reasonable to perform several smaller incisional biopsies at areas of highest suspicion within the larger lesion. Incisional biopsies should be designed to extend into clinically normal skin because this assists the pathologist in the evaluation and interpretation of the specimen.

Lesions that have been confirmed as LM should be treated as melanoma in situ. Given higher recurrence rates in nonsurgical treatment modalities (cryotherapy, laser therapy, radiation therapy, immunotherapy),[6-10] surgical excision is the treatment of choice.[11,12] Surgical options include standard excision with 5- to 10-mm clinical margins (National Comprehensive Cancer Network guidelines)[13] and staged excision with delayed closure.

LM lesions can have extensive subclinical extension (see Figure 22-1). Because of this, routine standard excisions of LM with 5 mm margins result in positive margins in 8% to 20% of cases.[14] To achieve histologically negative margins, techniques for more complete histologic evaluation of surgical margins should be considered. This is especially important in areas where functional considerations may render extirpation of the full 5-mm clinical margins difficult (see Figure 22-2). Recurrence, when it occurs, may present with more invasive disease. About 23% of patients with MIS left at the margin progress to invasive disease with an average Breslow depth of 0.94 mm.[15] A study of 1120 MIS determined that 6-mm margins had an 86% clearance rate and 9-mm margins had a 98.9% clearance rate.[16]

Staged excision with postoperative margin evaluation allows confirmation of clear margins prior to surgical repair. Margin evaluation is often performed *en face* instead of the usual bread-loafing. The benefits of staged excision with delayed reconstruction include a lower recurrence rate (5%)[17] and potential to change management prior to final reconstruction. For example, if the LM is found to have an invasive component, the surgeon can take a wider margin and/or consider sentinel lymph node biopsy and adjuvant therapy.

The use of Mohs surgery is controversial and many recommend against it given the inherent difficulty in assessing melanocytes in frozen section specimens. However, if augmented with immunoperoxidase stains or rush permanent sections, it may be a reasonable consideration.[18-20] Recent studies, including a large prospective series using variations of the Mohs procedure (eg, mapped serial excision, Slow-Mohs), have reported high early cure rates and tissue conservation in the setting of periocular melanoma.[21-23] Debulking of the gross clinical lesion is performed to assess for invasive disease and between 5% to 20% of the cases are upstaged to invasive melanoma.[24]

Imiquimod 5% cream has been used as immunotherapy for LM. A prospective analysis of 23 patients treated for 12 weeks showed 1 recurrence after a mean of 39 months of follow-up.[25] However, there have been reports of invasive disease developing during imiquimod treatment for LM, and evidence that clinical improvement in pigmentation does not necessarily correlate with histologic clearance.[9] Based on the current evidence, imiquimod may be a reasonable treatment option in poor surgical candidates or as an adjunct to surgical excision.

Radiation therapy is a reasonable choice for patients who are not operative candidates. The largest series to date followed up with 150 patients for a minimum of 2 years after treatment. Mean time to recurrence was 45 months, and the recurrence rate was 7%.[10]

Summary

LM is generally accepted as a form of MIS that occurs on chronically sun-damaged skin. A small subset will progress to invasive LMM. Excisional biopsy of the suspicious lesion is preferred, if feasible. Surgical treatment with a minimum of 5-mm clinical margins will result in positive margins in a fraction of cases. If possible, techniques for more thorough evaluation of histologic margins should be employed prior to reconstruction. In nonsurgical candidates, radiation and imiquimod may be of benefit.

References

1. Cohen LM. Lentigo maligna and lentigo maligna melanoma. *J Am Acad Dermatol.* 1995;33(6):923-936.
2. Weinstock MA, Sober AJ. The risk of progression of lentigo maligna to lentigo maligna melanoma. *Br J Dermatol.* 1987;116(3):303-310.
3. Agarwal-Antal N, Bowen GM, Gerwels JW. Histologic evaluation of lentigo maligna with permanent sections: implications regarding current guidelines. *J Am Acad Dermatol.* 2002;47:743-748.
4. Barnhill RL, Mihm MC Jr. The histopathology of cutaneous malignant melanoma. *Semin Diagn Pathol.* 1993;10:47-75.
5. Guitera P, Moloney FJ, Menzies SW, et al. Improving management and patient care in lentigo maligna by mapping with in vivo confocal microscopy. *JAMA Dermatol.* 2013;149(6):692-698.

6. Pitman GH, Kopf AW, Bart RS, Casson PR. Treatment of lentigo maligna and lentigo maligna melanoma. *J Dermatol Surg Oncol.* 1979;5(9):727-737.

7. McKenna JK, Florell SR, Goldman GD, Bowen GM. Lentigo maligna/lentigo maligna melanoma: current state of diagnosis and treatment. *Dermatol Surg.* 2006;32(4):493-504.

8. Madan V, August PJ. Lentigo maligna—outcomes of treatment with Q-switched Nd:YAG and alexandrite lasers. *Dermatol Surg.* 2009;35(4):607-611.

9. Junkins-Hopkins JM. Imiquimod use in the treatment of lentigo maligna. *J Am Acad Dermatol.* 2009;61(5):865-867.

10. Farshad A, Burg G, Panizzon R, Dummer R. A retrospective study of 150 patients with lentigo maligna and lentigo maligna melanoma and the efficacy of radiotherapy using Grenz or soft X-rays. *Br J Dermatol.* 2002;146(6):1042-1046.

11. Zalaudek I, Horn M, Richtig E. Local recurrence in melanoma in situ: influence of sex, age, site of involvement and therapeutic modalities. *Br J Dermatol.* 2003;148:703-708.

12. Clark GS, Pappas-Politis EC, Cherpelis BS, et al. Surgical management of melanoma in situ on chronically sun-damaged skin. *Cancer Control.* 2008;15(3):216-224.

13. Houghton A, Coit D, Bloomer W, et al. NCCN melanoma practice guidelines. National Comprehensive Cancer Network. *Oncology.* 1998;12(7A):153-177.

14. Osborne JE, Hutchinson PE. A follow-up study to investigate the efficacy of initial treatment of lentigo maligna with surgical excision. *Br J Plast Surg.* 2002;55:611-615.

15. Hui AM, Jacobson M, Markowitz O, Brooks NA, Siegel DM. Mohs micrographic surgery for the treatment of melanoma. *Dermatol Clin.* 2012;30(3):503-515.

16. Kunishige JH, Brodland DG, Zitelli JA. Surgical margins for melanoma in situ. *J Am Acad Dermatol.* 2012;66(3):438-444.

17. Bub JL, Berg D, Slee A, Odland PB. Management of lentigo maligna and lentigo maligna melanoma with staged excision: a 5-year follow-up. *Arch Dermatol.* 2004;140(5):552-558.

18. Bene NI, Healy C, Coldiron BM. Mohs micrographic surgery is accurate 95.1% of the time for melanoma in situ: a prospective study of 167 cases. *Dermatol Surg.* 2008;34(5):660-664.

19. Zalla MJ, Lim KK, Dicaudo DJ, Gagnot MM. Mohs micrographic excision of melanoma using immunostains. *Dermatol Surg.* 2000;26:771-784.

20. Cohen LM, McCall MW, Hodge SJ, Freedman JD, Callen JP, Zax RH. Successful treatment of lentigo maligna and lentigo maligna melanoma with Mohs' micrographic surgery aided by rush permanent sections. *Cancer.* 1994;73(12):2964-2970.

21. Shumaker PR, Kelley B, Swann MH, Greenway HT Jr. Modified Mohs micrographic surgery for periocular melanoma and melanoma in situ: long-term experience at Scripps Clinic. *Dermatol Surg.* 2009;35(8):1263-1270.

22. Then SY, Malhotra R, Barlow R, et al. Early cure rates with narrow-margin slow-Mohs surgery for periocular malignant melanoma. *Dermatol Surg.* 2009;35(1):17-23.

23. Malhotra R, Chen C, Huilgol SC, Hill DC, Selva D. Mapped serial excision for periocular lentigo maligna and lentigo maligna melanoma. *Ophthalmology.* 2003;110(10):2011-2018.

24. Iorizzo LJ 3rd, Chocron I, Lumbang W, Stasko T. Importance of vertical pathology of debulking specimens during Mohs micrographic surgery for lentigo maligna and melanoma in situ. *Dermatol Surg.* 2013;39(3 Pt 1):365-371.

25. Kirtschig G, van Meurs T, van Doorn R. Twelve-week treatment of lentigo maligna with imiquimod results in a high and sustained clearance rate. *Acta Derm Venereol.* 2015;95(1):83-85.

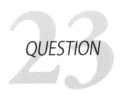
WHAT TOPICAL THERAPY CAN I USE TO TREAT CUTANEOUS MALIGNANCIES?

Heidi M. Hermes, MD, FAAD and
Timothy S. Wang, MD

It seems like we're moving toward less invasive management of many diseases. Is this true for skin cancer? What is your experience? Should I offer this to my patients or is it still in the development phase?

The most common cutaneous malignancies are basal cell and squamous cell carcinomas (BCC and SCC). Together, these are referred to as non-melanoma skin cancer (NMSC) and they frequently occur on the face and periocular region.[1] Actinic keratoses (AKs) are also highly prevalent on the face and represent precursors to cutaneous SCC. They carry a 4-year risk for transformation into SCC of up to 2.6%[2] and are thus often treated to prevent this transformation. Other less common but significant skin cancers found on the face include lentigo maligna (LM), lentigo maligna melanoma (LMM), Merkel cell, and sebaceous carcinoma.

The current standard of care for the treatment of NMSCs on the head and neck is surgical excision with margin control, either by standard excision with frozen section control or Mohs micrographic surgery (see Question 19). In patients unable to tolerate or who refuse surgery, radiotherapy (RT) is also a proven option. Interest in other nonsurgical options for the treatment of cutaneous malignancies on the face is high due to patients' desire to avoid a surgical scar. Food and Drug Administration (FDA) approval of topical therapies to treat superficial BCCs on the trunk and extremities has prompted investigation to broaden their use to include other locations and histologic growth patterns. It should be noted, however, that at the time of this writing, no topical therapy is FDA approved for the treatment of skin cancer on the face, and no topical therapy has been approved for the treatment of any type of skin cancers other than superficial growth pattern BCCs.

Available topical therapies vary in their mechanism of action as well as FDA approved indications and dosing regimens (Table 23-1). All are patient administered and share common drawbacks of poor margin control, protracted inflammation and irritation beyond clinical borders, lengthy course of treatment, and lower cure rates. Data for off-label use are limited, and typically reported as case reports or small case series with variable follow-up. Side effects of these therapies are summarized in Table 23-2.

Kersten RC, McCulley TJ, eds. *Curbside Consultation in Oculoplastics:*
49 Clinical Questions, Second Edition (pp 113-117).
© 2016 Taylor & Francis Group.

Table 23-1

Summary of Topical Therapies, Indication, Dosing Regimen, and Reported Clearance Rates

	Indication (dosage)	Regimen	Aggregated Clearance rates[1,2]
Imiquimod			
On Label	Thin AKs on face and scalp (5%, 3.75%, 2.5%)	Twice weekly for 16 weeks or nightly for 2 weeks	60%
	Superficial BCC on neck, body, and extremity (5%)	5 times weekly for 6 weeks	80%
Off Label	Other BCC subtypes		65%
	SCC in situ		76%
	Lentigo maligna		53%
5-fluorouracil			
On Label	AKs (5%, 2%, 0.5%)	Twice a day for 2 to 4 weeks	82%
	Superficial BCC on the body or extremity (5%)	Twice a day for 4 to 6 weeks	92%
Off Label	SCC in situ		61%
Ingenol Mebutate			
On Label	AK on the face and scalp (0.015%)	3 consecutive days	64%
	AK on the body and extremity (0.05%)	2 consecutive days	50%
Off Label	Superficial BCC		63%
Diclofenac			
On Label	AKs (3%)	Twice a day for 60 to 90 days	30% to 40%

AKs = actinic keratoses; BCC = basal cell carcinoma; SCC = squamous cell carcinoma.
1. Clearance rates for AKs are for partial clearance rates (>75% clinical clearance at endpoint).
2. Clearance rates for cutaneous malignancies are reported as clinical clearance at endpoint.
Adapted from Chitwood K, Etzkorn J, Cohen G. Topical and intralesional treatment of nonmelanoma skin cancer: efficacy and cost comparisons. *Dermatol Surg.* 2013;39(9):1306-1316.

Table 23-2
Summary of Side Effects Encountered With Topical Regimens

Topical Regimen	*Side Effect(s)*
Imiquimod	Common: erythema, erosions
	Rare: systemic flu-like symptoms, urinary retention
	Ocular: conjunctivitis, keratitis, preseptal cellulitis
5-fluorouricil	Common: erythema, prurritus, photosensitivity
	Rare: systemic toxicity—caution in DPD deficient patients
	Ocular: keratopathy
Ingenol Mebutate	Common: erythema, scaling
Diclofenac	Common: mild erythema
	Rare: systemic absorption, anaphylaxis in NSAID-sensitive patients
Tazarotine	Common: erythema, scaling

DPD = dihydropyrimidine dehydrogenase; NSAID = nonsteroidal anti-inflammatory drug.

Imiquimod (Aldara 5% cream, Zyclara 2.5% or 3.75% cream, generic 5% cream) is an immune modulator that stimulates the innate immune system via toll-like receptors (TLR) 7 and 8. This purportedly induces proinflammatory cytokines producing antitumor responses. Original FDA approval was granted in 1997 for the 5% cream treatment of thin actinic keratoses (AKs) of the face and scalp, used twice weekly for 16 weeks. Subsequent formulations of 2.5% and 3.75% have been released, again approved for actinic keratosis on the face and scalp, and administered nightly for 2 weeks. In 2004, imiquimod 5% was approved for the treatment of superficial BCCs less than 2 cm in diameter occurring on the neck, body, or extremity. The regimen is 5 times per week for 6 weeks, achieving clinical clearance rates of about 80%. Off-label use for this formulation on other histologic BCC subtypes (specifically nodular BCCs) have been reported to be around 65%.[3] Aggregate clearance rates using imiquimod for SCC in situ (SCCis) are about 76%[3] and 53% for lentigo maligna.[1] Several case reports have described imiquimod use for periorbital BCC of various histologic subtypes with 80% clearance rate, and one case report of complete clearance of SCCis.[4] Adverse effects are mainly local inflammatory reactions such as erythema and erosions. Conjunctivitis, keratitis, and preseptal cellulitis have been described with periocular use[5] (Figure 23-1). Rarely, systemic symptoms such as a flu-like reaction or urinary retention can occur. The inflammatory reaction typically resolves in 2 to 3 weeks upon discontinuation of the medication.[5] Imiquimod is also approved for treatment of external genital warts, a point worth disclosing to patients to avoid confusion.

The pyrimidine analog 5-fluorouracil (5FU) (Efudex 5% cream, Fluoroplex 1% cream, Carac 0.5% cream, generic 5% cream, generic 5% or 2% solution) acts as an antimetabolite, depleting the cell of thymidine and decreasing DNA synthesis, which leads to cell death. Cells with rapid turnover such as precancerous and tumor cells are particularly susceptible. The 5% topical formu-

Figure 23-1. Periocular inflammatory response with mild conjunctivitis following imiquimod treatment. (Reprinted with permission from Murchison AP, Walrath JD, Washington CV. Non-surgical treatments of primary, non-melanoma eyelid malignancies: a review. *Clin Experiment Ophthalmol.* 2011;39(1):65-83. © 2011 John Wiley and Sons.)

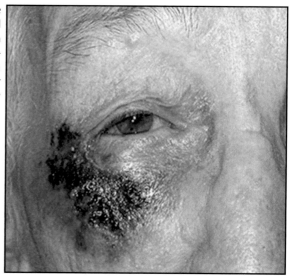

lation was FDA approved in the 1970s and is currently indicated for the treatment of AKs and superficial BCCs on the body or extremities. Use is twice daily for 2 to 4 weeks for AKs and up to 6 weeks for superficial BCCs. Clearance rates for superficial BCCs are reportedly as high as 92%, but there have been reports of histologic persistence despite apparent clinical cure.[6] Off-label use for treating SCCis affords lower cure rates averaging 61%.[3] The lower concentration formulations are approved for AKs on the head and neck with the same dosing schedule. Use is generally titrated to effect, with the most common effects being erythema, prutitus, and photosensitivity. Keratopathy is the most common ocular side effect.[5] Systemic toxicity is rare. The enzyme dihydropyrimidine dehydrogenase (DPD) metabolizes 5FU and an exaggerated response may be seen in DPD deficient patients.

There are several other classes of topical therapies commonly used as field therapy or adjuvant treatment for AKs. Ingenol mebutate (Picato 0.05% and 0.015% gel) is a macrocyclic diterpene ester derived from sap of the Euphorbia peplus plant. It induces primary cell necrosis and cellular toxicity pathways via protein kinase C activation. It was approved in 2012 by the FDA for treatment of AKs. There are two concentrations and regimens: the 0.015% gel is for AKs on the face and scalp for 3 consecutive days and the 0.05% formulation for 2 consecutive days on the body or extremities. Preliminary results from the phase II trial for treatment of superficial BCC with the 0.05% formula showed 63% clearance.[6] Other off-label studies are ongoing, but currently there is insufficient evidence to support use for the treatment of NMSC. Adverse effects are erythema and scaling, and these are seen in over two-thirds of patients. Diclofenac topical is a nonspecific cyclooxygenase (COX) inhibitor, nonsteroidal anti-inflammatory drug (NSAID). Despite multiple topical formulations, the 3% gel (Solaraze) is the only one FDA approved for the treatment of AKs. It is a twice-daily application for 60 to 90 days. Clearance rates for AKs range between 30% and 40%.[6] Data on its use in NMSC are limited, as other topical medications have proved more effective. Adverse events are mild, but with prolonged use include systemic absorption and possible anaphylactic reactions in NSAID-sensitive patients. Topical retinoids such as tretinoin (multiple formulations, 0.1%, 0.05% and 0.025% cream or gel) or tazarotine (Tazorac 0.1%, 0.05% gel) are not FDA approved for the treatment of precancerous or cutaneous malignancies. Retinoids bind retinoid receptors in the cell nucleus, and have downstream effects regulating cell proliferation and apoptosis.[7] They are sometimes employed as adjuvant therapy to enhance epidermal penetration of other topical medications. Studies evaluating topical retinoid use as chemoprevention for cutaneous malignancies have been disappointing.

Summary

For NMSC on the head and neck, surgical excision remains the standard of therapy. In nonsurgical candidates or those who refuse surgery, radiation therapy is an accepted option. Some topical therapies are approved for low-risk superficial BCCs on the trunk and extremities; however, their use to treat cutaneous malignancies on the head and neck remains off-label. Additional barriers to topical therapy use on the face and periocular locations include prolonged course of treatment (often 6 to 8 weeks), high frequency of inflammatory side effects, reducing patient compliance, and unproven efficacy. Risks, benefits, and discussion about off-label use should be thoroughly explored with each individual patient.

References

1. Slutsky JB, Jones EC. Periocular cutaneous malignancies: a review of the literature. *Dermatol Surg.* 2012;38(4):552-569.
2. Criscione VD, Weinstock MA, Naylor MF, et al. Actinic keratoses. *Cancer.* 2009;115(11):2523-2530.
3. Chitwood K, Etzkorn J, Cohen G. Topical and intralesional treatment of nonmelanoma skin cancer: efficacy and cost comparisons. *Dermatol Surg.* 2013;39(9):1306-1316.
4. Brannan PA, Anderson HK, Kersten RC, Kulwin DR. Bowen disease of the eyelid successfully treated with imiquimod. *Ophthal Plast Reconstr Surg.* 2005;21(4):321-322.
5. Sullivan TJ. Topical therapies for periorbital cutaneous malignancies: indications and treatment regimens. *Curr Opin Ophthalmol.* 2012;23(5):439-442.
6. Bahner JD, Bordeaux JS. Non-melanoma skin cancers: photodynamic therapy, cryotherapy, 5-fluorouracil, Imiquimod, Diclofenac, or what? Facts and controversies. *Clin Dermatol.* 2013;31(6):792-798.
7. Murchison AP, Walrath JD, Washington CV. Non-surgical treatments of primary, non-melanoma eyelid malignancies: a review. *Clin Experiment Ophthalmol.* 2011;39(1):65,83; quiz 92-3.

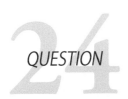

WHAT SYSTEMIC MEDICAL THERAPY IS AVAILABLE FOR TREATMENT OF CUTANEOUS MALIGNANCIES?

Bobby S. Korn, MD, PhD and
Bradford Lee, MD, MSc

When do you consider systemic medical therapy for skin cancer? What agents are available, and what role do they play in your practice?

Basal cell carcinoma (BCC) and squamous cell carcinoma (SCC) represent the vast majority of cutaneous malignancies of the eyelid and periocular region. In most cases, BCC and SCC lesions can be excised surgically with intraoperative frozen margins or Mohs micrographic surgery. Once margin clearance has been achieved, surgical reconstruction is initiated.

Although surgical excision remains the gold standard of therapy, certain factors may make surgical excision a suboptimal or even undesirable therapeutic option. The physician must consider the patient as a whole, including the patient's global comorbidities, life expectancy, and degree of morbidity associated with complete excision with reconstruction. Some factors to consider include the following:

- Metastatic disease
- Orbital invasion involving vital orbital structures
- Monocular status
- Locally advanced disease
- Perineural invasion (eg, around the facial nerve)
- Unusually high risk for subsequent malignancies (eg, Gorlin-Goltz syndrome)
- Patient comorbidities impacting surgical candidacy
- Patient life expectancy

Although not the focus of this chapter, other nonsystemic therapies should also be considered such as curettage, electrocautery, cryotherapy, topical 5-fluorouracil, photodynamic therapy, and local immunomodulatory therapies such as imiquimod.

Kersten RC, McCulley TJ, eds. *Curbside Consultation in Oculoplastics:*
49 Clinical Questions, Second Edition (pp 119-121).
© 2016 Taylor & Francis Group.

The number of systemic therapies available and in clinical trials is prodigious and constantly changing. Here, we will focus on several of the most important and efficacious systemic therapies currently available for treatment of BCC and SCC.

Basal Cell Carcinoma

A critical cell-signaling pathway in BCC is the hedgehog pathway, whose inappropriate activation leads to abnormal proliferation of basal cells. Molecular studies have found that the majority of BCC carry either a loss of function mutation in the tumor suppressor gene PTCH1 or gain of function mutation in smoothened, both of which are involved in the hedgehog cell signaling pathway.

Vismodegib was approved by the FDA in January 2012 and is the first oral small-molecule inhibitor of the Hedgehog pathway. Its indication is for locally advanced or metastatic BCC and has been found to be effective in basal cell nevus syndrome (Gorlin-Goltz syndrome). It is also indicated for BCC in patients who are poor surgical or radiotherapy candidates. A Phase I study of vismodegib demonstrated a 58% response rate among patients with advanced BCC. A Phase II study showed a 30% response rate in patients with metastatic BCC and a 43% response rate in patients with locally advanced BCC (21% complete response rate). Median duration of response was 7.6 months for both cohorts, and common adverse events included muscle spasms, alopecia, distortion of sense of taste, weight loss, and fatigue.[1] Administration during pregnancy is contraindicated because of the embryotoxic and teratogenic effects in animal studies.

Kahana et al reported on the use of vismodegib in a patient with BCC invading the medial orbit for whom total excision would have required exenteration with loss of the eye.[2] Neoadjuvant vismodegib treatment was used for 4 months, resulting in tumor shrinkage. Eventually, globe-sparing en bloc excision of the residual orbital mass was performed.

Gill et al reported the use of vismodegib in 7 patients with infiltrative BCC not amenable to surgery or radiation.[3] All patients demonstrated varying degrees of regression of the carcinoma, with 2 of the patients showing complete clinical regression. Interestingly, 2 of these patients developed new SCCs at distinct clinical sites. Whether this was a consequence of treatment or an unrelated occurrence is unknown. Second-site recurrence of malignant skin tumors has not been reported with vismodegib prior to this study. This phenomenon is not unknown, as patients on other antitumor agents have been reported to develop second-site malignancies. Expanded use of vismodegib will yield further information on this potential interaction.

Squamous Cell Carcinoma

Isolated, periorbital, and eyelid SCC are treated in a similar fashion to BCC. However, compared to BCC, SCC has a higher tendency for local spread through perineural invasion. In advanced cases of orbital invasion, radical surgery including orbital exenteration and adjunctive radiotherapy may be required. Molecular targeted therapies may be considered in such advanced cases of SCC.

The epidermal growth factor receptor (EGFR) is highly expressed in SCC, and increased EGFR signaling has been associated with aggressive disease, metastatic SCC, and overall poor prognosis.[4] Cetuximab is a monoclonal antibody against EGFR that is approved for SCC of the head and neck. It works via multiple mechanisms in slowing proliferation, inducing apoptosis, and inhibiting angiogenesis. There have been various reports of clinical response to cetuximab in patients with recurrent or metastatic SCC, both as monotherapy as well as in combination with platinum-containing chemotherapeutics.[5,6]

EGFR tyrosine kinase inhibitors (TKIs) represent another class of small molecules that suppress cell signaling via the EGFR's intracellular tyrosine kinase domain. There have been reports and Phase II trials demonstrating the efficacy of gefitinib and erlotinib in achieving disease stability, partial response, or complete response for unresectable cutaneous SCC.[7,8] El-Sawy et al reported 2 cases of locally invasive SCC into the orbit that were treated with either cetuximab or erlotinib and resulted in marked clinical and radiological improvement.[9]

Summary

Surgical resection remains the standard of care for periocular BCC and SCC whenever margins can be obtained in patients fit for surgery. However, in the setting of unresectable lesions, metastatic lesions, or lesions whose resection would result in loss of vital structures such as the globe or the facial nerve, systemic small molecule therapies may be considered as new and potentially promising options, whether as neoadjuvant therapy, adjuvant therapy, monotherapy, or in combination with other nonsurgical treatments.

References

1. Sekulic A, Migden MR, Oro AE, et al. Efficacy and safety of vismodegib in advanced basal-cell carcinoma. *N Engl J Med*. 2012;366(23):2171-2179.
2. Kahana A, Worden FP, Elner VM. Vismodegib as eye-sparing adjuvant treatment for orbital basal cell carcinoma. *JAMA Ophthalmol*. 2013;131(10):1364-1366.
3. Gill HS, Moscato EE, Chang ALS, Soon S, Silkiss RZ. Vismodegib for periocular and orbital basal cell carcinoma. *JAMA Ophthalmol*. 2013;131(12):1591-1594.
4. Shimizu T, Izumi H, Oga A, et al. Epidermal growth factor receptor overexpression and genetic aberrations in metastatic squamous cell carcinoma of the skin. *Dermatology*. 2001;202:203-206.
5. Burtness B. The role of cetuximab in the treatment of squamous cell cancer of the head and neck. *Expert Opin Biol Ther*. 2005;5(8):1085-1093.
6. Vega-Villegas E, Awada R, Mesia L, et al. A phase I study of cetuximab in combination with cisplatin or carboplatin and 5-FU in patients with recurrent or metastatic squamous cell carcinoma of the head and neck. *Proc Am Assoc Cancer Res*. 2003;22:2020.
7. Glisson BS, Kim ES, Kies MS, et al. Phase II study of gefitinib in patients with metastatic/recurrent squamous cell carcinoma of the skin. *J Clin Oncol (Meeting Abstracts)*. 2006;24(18 suppl) Abstract 5531.
8. Cranmer LD, Engelhardt C, Morgan SS. Treatment of unresectable and metastatic cutaneous squamous cell carcinoma. *Oncologist*. 2010;15(12):1320-1328.
9. El-Sawy T, Sabichi AL, Myers JN, et al. Epidermal growth factor receptor inhibitors for treatment of orbital squamous cell carcinoma. *Arch Ophthalmol*. 2012;130(12):1608-1611.

SECTION III

ORBITAL DISEASE

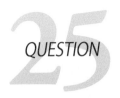

How Do I Know When To Order MRI or CT?

Karl C. Golnik, MD, MEd

How do magnetic resonance imaging (MRI) and computed tomography (CT) work? When should I order an MRI and when is CT preferred, or at least adequate? When is either contraindicated?

Practitioners are often faced with selecting the correct neuroimaging modality. Most commonly, you must decide between a CT scan and an MRI. Figures 25-1 and 25-2 demonstrate the potential usefulness of both. The choice depends on a variety of factors, including suspected diagnosis, anatomic location of suspected abnormality, availability of imaging modality, and cost.

Sometimes, patient factors unrelated to the diagnosis in question preclude obtaining one or the other type of study, thus obviating your decision-making process. The presence of ferromagnetic material within the body (eg, cardiac pacemaker) precludes MRI. Recent intra-arterial stent placement (within the past 6 months) is thought to be a relative contraindication to MRI. Severe claustrophobia may prevent obtaining any form of MRI. Moderate claustrophobia may be overcome by antianxiety drug administration or performing an open MRI. Finally, some patients with severe scoliosis or congestive heart failure cannot lie flat and neither conventional CT scan or MRI can be obtained. Larger cities may have standing/sitting MRI centers that will allow study of these patients.

Fortunately, the majority of patients do not have contraindications regarding the type of imaging that is ordered. Table 25-1 provides a loose framework for choosing MRI or CT for some more commonly encountered abnormalities. In general, MRI is better for investigating probable brain and skull base processes, and is equivalent to CT scan for primary orbital processes. CT scan is superior for bone evaluation and for differentiating between calcification and other tissues. Therefore, if you are fairly certain that the abnormality is orbital (eg, thyroid eye disease), then orbital CT scan is adequate. However, if you are not sure, or if there is an entity in the differential diagnosis that might extend intracranially, then MRI is superior. MRI is the best choice for

Kersten RC, McCulley TJ, eds. *Curbside Consultation in Oculoplastics: 49 Clinical Questions, Second Edition* (pp 125-128). © 2016 Taylor & Francis Group.

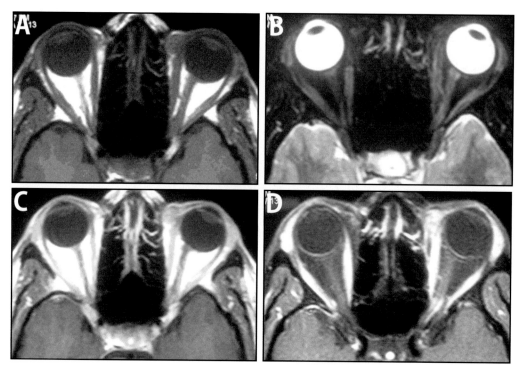

Figure 25-1. Magnetic resonance imaging. All MR images are from the same patient who has a left orbital apex optic nerve sheath meningioma. (A) MRI T1 axial image through the mid-orbit. Note bright white orbital fat signal. On T1 images, water (vitreous) appears black. (B) MRI T2 fat suppressed image through the mid-orbit. Note the lack of white fat signal. On T2 signals, water (vitreous) appears white. The optic nerve sheath meningioma is not readily apparent. (C) MRI T1 postgadolinium, nonfat suppressed image. No definite gadolinium enhancement of the optic nerve is noted. The fat signal obscures the adjacent enhancement of the meningioma. (D) MRI T1 postgadolinium image with fat suppression. Note the tram-track-like enhancement of the posterior orbital optic nerve, indicating optic nerve sheath meningioma.

unexplained suspected optic neuropathy because you want to get a good look at the whole optic nerve. Bones or calcification are not well visualized on MRI, thus if you are interested in bony detail or the presence of calcification (eg, fracture, bone erosion), a CT scan should be ordered.

Blood vessels can be imaged by MRI because the moving protons in blood preclude obtaining a summed signal, thus one sees a flow void where the vessel is located. Of course, if you are specifically interested in blood vessels (eg, aneurysm, cavernous sinus fistula), magnetic resonance angiography (MRA) can be obtained at the same time as the MRI by using different computer software. Contrast administration can be used in MRA, but it is not essential. Computed tomographic angiography (CTA) has gained acceptance as an alternate method for vascular evaluation. The study duration is shorter, but contrast must be given. Local availability and expert interpretation of these imaging techniques may vary and must be part of your decision-making process. Relative availability may also be a factor if there is perceived urgency based on the potential underlying abnormality. Finally, a CT scan generally costs much less than MRI and therefore a CT scan should be ordered if it has equal (or better) utility. If repeated imaging is required, one must consider radiation exposure with repeated CT scans, especially in young children.

Table 25-2 outlines some general guidelines to use when ordering orbital imaging studies. There are a couple of important technical points to mention. Although most centers perform direct coronal images when orbital CT is ordered, I always request direct coronal images because this is not routine in every center. However, newer multiport spiral-CT scanners rapidly scan in a

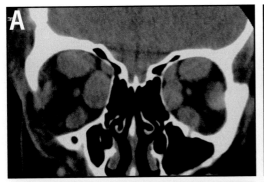
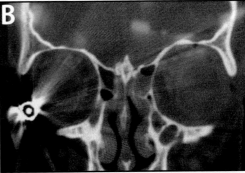
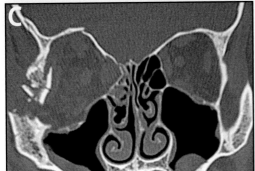

Figure 25-2. Computed tomography. (A) The characteristic findings of thyroid eye disease are readily appreciable with CT. (B) CT is the preferred modality to locate metallic foreign bodies. A bullet is seen in the right orbit of this patient. (C) Fractures, such as the tripod fracture in this patient, are best assessed with CT.

Table 25-1

Indications for Magnetic Resonance Imaging and Computed Tomography

MRI is far superior	Intracranial malignancy Stroke
MRI in most cases is superior	Orbital neoplasm Orbital or periocular pain
CT is superior (or at least adequate)	Thyroid eye disease Orbital fracture Metallic foreign bodies

MRI = magnetic resonance imaging; CT = computed tomography

helical fashion and allow excellent coronal, sagittal, and axial resolution. Additionally, if an MRI is ordered of the brain (not orbits), you may not get coronal images through the orbits. Often, ordering brain MRI with attention to the orbits will give you the necessary information without producing bills for two separate MRIs. Finally, when ordering an MRI, it is crucial to obtain fat-suppressed images when evaluating the orbits. This eliminates the bright white fat signal that

Table 25-2

General Specifications Used When Ordering Orbital Imaging Studies

Modality	Computed Tomography	Magnetic Resonance Imaging
"Cut Size"	Fine cuts (1 mm preferably) (3 mm is usually adequate)	Fine cuts (same as CT)
Plane	Axial and "direct" coronal	Axial, coronal, and sagittal
Contrast	With and without contrast*	With and without contrast**

CT = computed tomography
* When assessing patients for an orbital fracture, contrast is not needed.
** When neoplasm is suspected, specify that T1 fat-suppressed images with and without contrast are included.

might obscure intraorbital abnormalities (see Figures 25-1A and B). Fat suppression usually will not be done if the MRI is ordered of the brain alone.

Contrast administration is almost always desirable (see Figures 25-1B to D). Exceptions include scans for known thyroid eye disease, bone evaluation, and differentiating calcification from blood. Of course, the presence of allergy may affect the choice of imaging. Allergy to iodine precludes CT scan dye administration. Rarely, gadolinium allergy precludes administration for MRI. Renal dysfunction may preclude the use of any contrast material.

My final advice is that if you are still unsure about what type of imaging to order, call a good neuroradiologist and explain the diagnostic possibilities. He or she should be able to guide you to the correct neuroimaging study.

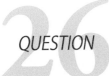

WHAT IS IGG4 IMMUNE-RELATED INFLAMMATION OF THE ORBIT AND HOW DO YOU TREAT IT?

Elizabeth A. Atchison, MD and
James A. Garrity, MD

I recently saw a patient who had been treated for IgG4 immune-related inflammation. Is this different from other forms of orbital inflammation? Does this diagnosis affect prognosis or management?

Immunoglobin G4–related diseases (IgG4-RD) are a relatively new recognized category of diseases characterized by fibrosing inflammation accompanied by IgG4 positive plasma cells. The family of IgG immunoglobulins is comprised of 4 subclasses (IgG1-4), with IgG4 being the least common of the 4 subtypes. It is a functionally monovalent antibody and is not able to activate the classic complement pathway as do the other subtypes. IgG4 levels tend to be elevated in allergic diseases and with chronic antigen stimulation. IgG4-RD was originally recognized in the context of autoimmune pancreatitis, and was subsequently identified as a syndrome affecting many body systems, including the orbit. The organs most commonly affected are the pancreas, hepatobiliary system, salivary glands, lymph nodes, and orbits. Twenty percent of those with IgG4-RD will have involvement of the head or neck, and of those, 43% will have involvement of the orbit.[1]

There are many possible presentations of IgG4-RD of the orbit and a common theme is an absence of the typical features of inflammation, notably pain and erythema. The first description of orbital disease was lacrimal gland enlargement, which was typically bilateral and longstanding. As more patients have been diagnosed with IgG4-RD, involvement of other orbital structures has been noted. The diagnosis is slightly more common in men, with an average age of 50 at diagnosis, but can present at any age in either gender.[2,3] Most patients, regardless of which orbital structure is involved, present with painless mass lesions. The few patients we have seen with pain had soft tissue infiltrates near their trochlea and probably experienced trochlear headaches on this basis. Because of the tendency of IgG4-RD to form tumefactive lesions, it often raises initial concern for malignancy, especially lymphoma given the notable lack of symptoms despite the mass evident on neuroimaging. Most with orbital involvement have bilateral disease and some systemic

Kersten RC, McCulley TJ, eds. *Curbside Consultation in Oculoplastics:*
49 Clinical Questions, Second Edition (pp 129-132).
© 2016 Taylor & Francis Group.

Table 26-1
Radiographic Findings in 27 Patients With Biopsy-Proven IgG4-RD

Extraocular Muscles	*89%*
Bilateral	88%
Lateral rectus	71%
Lacrimal Gland	*70%*
Bilateral	58%
Orbital Infiltrate	*44%*
Infraorbital Nerve Enlargement	*30%*
Bilateral	63%
Intracranial	*11%*
Cavernous Sinus Disease	100%
Sinus Disease	*89%*
Mild	30%
Moderate	40%
Marked	30%

involvement. When we compared 13 IgG4 positive patients with 8 IgG4 negative patients, we noted that 5 of the positive group had asthma, 4 had lymphadenopathy, and 3 had gastrointestinal disease (1 pseudotumor of liver, 1 biliary cirrhosis, 1 pancreatitis), while the negative group had 1 lymphadenopathy, 1 asthma, and 1 submandibular mucosa–associated lymphoid tissue (MALT) lymphoma.[2,4]

While it is still a valuable clinical rule that orbital involvement with multisystem disease should make the clinician think of granulomatosis with polyangiitis (formerly Wegener granulomatosis), the same can now be said for IgG4-RD, especially if asthma, retroperitoneal fibrosis, autoimmune pancreatitis, or other constitutional symptoms are present. Initial workup of these cases should include a thorough review of systems and past medical history to investigate other sites of IgG4-RD.

Radiographic findings on computed tomography (CT) and magnetic resonance imaging (MRI) are diverse and can include lacrimal gland enlargement, enlarged extraocular muscles, orbital soft tissue infiltrates, or enlarged infraorbital nerves. We have examined radiographic findings in 27 patients[5] with biopsy-proven IgG4-RD (Table 26-1). Extraocular muscle enlargement was the most frequent finding and can be confused with Graves' ophthalmopathy. Disproportionate enlargement of the lateral rectus muscle, however, is a clue to IgG4-RD because the lateral rectus muscle is the most frequently involved muscle in IgG4-RD. By contrast, the lateral rectus is only involved (and to a lesser extent) if the other rectus muscles are involved in Graves' ophthalmopathy. Another finding that appears to be characteristic of IgG4-RD is enlargement of the infraorbital nerve. In our experience, any other orbital finding in combination with an enlarged infraorbital nerve will prove to be IgG4-RD (Figure 26-1). An interesting finding regarding the

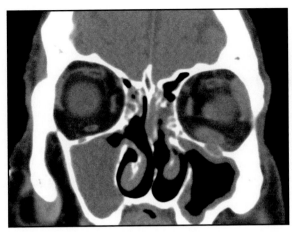

Figure 26-1. Coronal computed tomography scan of orbital IgG4-RD: Moderately severe membrane thickening within all the paranasal sinuses results in complete or near-complete opacification of right antrum. Enlargement of left inferior rectus, left lateral rectus (not shown), left lacrimal gland, and left infraorbital nerve. Right orbit was normal.

enlarged infraorbital nerve is that the nerve retains its function in contradistinction to an enlarged infraorbital nerve that is infiltrated with tumor. We have histologic findings on one infraorbital nerve biopsy and this shows Ig4 plasma cell infiltration of the peri- and epineuron. The endoneuron was spared. One must exercise caution in patients with orbital findings and sinus disease because granulomatosis with polyangiitis is a diagnostic possibility in this setting.

Diagnosis of IgG4-RD can sometimes be challenging. There are organ-specific diagnostic criteria proposed[6] but in general, the best way to diagnose IgG4-RD is with a biopsy. The first diagnostic criterion is the morphologic appearance of the biopsy. The second criterion is the presence of IgG4 staining plasma cells. The absolute number of IgG4 staining cells is noted. Some centers use 10 IgG4 positive cells per high power field (HPF), others use 30 per HPF, and others propose 50 per HPF. The ratio of positively staining cells divided by the number of IgG staining cells should be 40% or greater. Both IgG4 and IgG staining can be done off the paraffin blocks. An elevated serum IgG4 level of 135 or greater is further supporting evidence. There will be varying degrees of fibrosis, and as the amount of fibrosis increases, the absolute number of IgG4 staining cells may go down. As a cautionary note, we have noted that some patients with orbital granulomatosis with polyangiitis will stain positively for IgG4 and the ratio of IgG4-to-IgG is also elevated beyond 40%. This further emphasizes the role of morphologic appearance in establishing the diagnosis.[7]

Although there has been no causal association between the lymphoid hyperplasia of IgG4-RD and lymphoma, there have been some associations. One study noted 3 cases of lacrimal gland lymphoma arising within the context of IgG4-RD and 3 cases of lacrimal gland lymphoma that were IgG4 positive.[8] Another study looked at 114 cases of ocular adnexal marginal zone lymphomas and noted that 10 (9%) were IgG4 positive.[9] We have seen one lymphoma in association with IgG4-RD.

In terms of ancillary evaluation, we would suggest CT scanning of the chest and abdomen along with measurement of serum IgG4 level as screening tests. Further evaluation can be predicated upon results of this testing. Treatment has yet to be definitively outlined, but generally steroids, either high dose orally or injected intralesionally, are first line. Virtually all patients with IgG4-RD will respond to steroids, but problems may ensue with steroid dependency or drug-induced side effects. If the disease is confined to the orbit, a useful option is intralesional steroid injections as needed. It has been our practice to inject 40 mg triamcinolone and 4 mg dexamethasone at the time of incisional biopsy and then repeating as necessary. If the patient fails to respond to steroid therapy or recurs after taper then rituximab has been our second-line agent of choice. Other immunomodulatory agents have been tried with more limited success.[2] It is also interesting to note that in our patients we have only seen one associated lymphoma (1 of 27; 3.7%) while

2 other reports have described a nearly 10% rate. Most of our patients were treated with rituximab, which theoretically could preclude development of an associated lymphoma.

Summary

Patients with IgG4-RD often present with symptoms and signs suggestive of a lymphoma. Radiographic findings may show enlarged lacrimal glands or extraocular muscles (especially the lateral rectus muscles). Enlarged infraorbital nerves are very suggestive of IgG4-RD. Biopsy findings are often described as "reactive lymphoid hyperplasia" with varying degrees of fibrosis until IgG4 studies are done. Initial treatment typically involves steroids but often includes rituximab if steroids fail.

References

1. Zen Y, Nakanuma Y. IgG4-related disease: a cross-sectional study of 114 cases. *Am J Surg Pathol.* 2010;34(12):1812-1819.
2. Wallace ZS, Deshpande V, Stone JH. Ophthalmic manifestations of IgG4-related disease: single-center experience and literature review. *Semin Arthritis Rheum.* 2013;43(6):806-817.
3. Carruthers MN, Khosroshahi A, Augustin T, Deshpande V, Stone JH. The diagnostic utility of serum IgG4 concentrations in IgG4-related disease. *Ann Rheum Dis.* 2015;74(1):14-18.
4. Plaza JA, Garrity JA, Dogan A, Ananthamurthy A, Witzig TE, Salomão DR. Orbital inflammation with IgG4-positive plasma cells: manifestation of IgG4 systemic disease. *Arch Ophthalmol.* 2011;129(4):421-428.
5. Tiegs-Heiden CA, Eckel LJ, Hunt CH, et al. Immunoglobulin G4-related disease of the orbit: imaging features in 27 patients. *AJNR Am J Neuroradiol.* 2014;35(7):1393-1397.
6. Deshpande V, Zen Y, Chan JK, et al. Consensus statement on the pathology of IgG4-related disease. *Mod Pathol.* 2012;25(9):1181-1192.
7. Chang SY, Keogh KA, Lewis JE, et al. IgG4-positive plasma cells in granulomatosis with polyangiitis (Wegener's): a clinicopathologic and immunohistochemical study on 43 granulomatosis with polyangiitis and 20 control cases. *Hum Pathol.* 2013;44(11):2432-2437.
8. Cheuk W, Yuen HKL, Chan AC, et al. Ocular adnexal lymphoma associated with IgG4+ chronic sclerosing dacryoadenitis: a previously undescribed complication of IgG4-related sclerosing disease. *Am J Surg Pathol.* 2008;32(8):1159-1167.
9. Kubota T, Moritani S, Yoshino T, Nagai H, Terasaki H. Ocular adnexal marginal zone B cell lymphoma infiltrated by IgG4-positive plasma cells. *J Clin Pathol.* 2010;63(12):1059-1065.

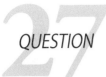
CAN YOU TELL ME ABOUT ORBITAL INFECTION DUE TO HOSPITAL- AND COMMUNITY-ACQUIRED MRSA?

Michael T. Yen, MD

Does it make any difference whether the bacteria came from home or the hospital? Do you ever recommend steroids for a patient with a bacterial infection?

The microbiology of orbital infections has dramatically changed over the past several decades.[1] With the widespread immunization of the population against organisms such as *Haemophilus influenza* B, the most common organisms now causing orbital cellulitis are *Staphylococcus* and *Streptococcus*. During this same period, many communities have seen a significant increase in the incidence of drug resistance, particularly with methicillin-resistant *Staphylococcus aureus* (MRSA), in both hospital- and community-acquired infections.[2] MRSA acquired in the community often differs from that encountered in the hospital. Although community-acquired MRSA tends to be sensitive to more antibiotics (less resistant), it is often more destructive. This relates to a specific toxic more often found in community-acquired strains that causes tissue destruction. There are tests available to distinguish community- and hospital-acquired strains, but I treat patients with maximal caution, regardless of where they caught the bug, so I don't usually request this.

There can also be significant variability in resistance rates in different communities. For example, in Houston the incidence of community-acquired MRSA infections has been reported to be >75%.[2] However, in Denver, the incidence of MRSA in orbital infections was reported to be about 12%.[3] Therefore, the successful management of orbital cellulitis requires suspicion for and knowledge about the level of MRSA activity in the hospital and community.

Over the past century, the introduction of antibiotic therapy and improvements in diagnostic technology and surgical techniques has greatly reduced the mortality and morbidity of orbital cellulitis.[4] However, management of orbital cellulitis continues to remain challenging. The medical management of orbital cellulitis requires aggressive antibiotic therapy as well as nasal treatments for the underlying sinusitis. Occasionally, such as with the presence of infected foreign bodies,

Kersten RC, McCulley TJ, eds. *Curbside Consultation in Oculoplastics:*
49 Clinical Questions, Second Edition (pp 133-136).
© 2016 Taylor & Francis Group.

immediate surgical intervention is clearly indicated. For cases of orbital cellulitis that develop an orbital abscess, the need for and timing of surgical intervention is less obvious. Adjunct intravenous corticosteroid therapy may be a beneficial treatment as well.[5] The successful management of orbital cellulitis may require a multidisciplinary approach with close communication between the ophthalmologist, otolaryngologist, neurosurgeon, radiologist, pediatrician, microbiologist, and infectious disease consultant.

Patients with MRSA orbital cellulitis present with the same clinical symptoms and signs as any other orbital infection. They usually present with severe eyelid edema associated with proptosis and pain with extraocular movements. There is often a history of an upper respiratory infection, nasal congestion, or acute sinusitis in the days preceding the development of eyelid edema. To promptly and accurately diagnose the condition, a systematic evaluation should be performed for all patients with a presentation suspicious for orbital cellulitis.

- Measure and document vital signs and constitutional symptoms. This includes the presence of fever, loss of appetite, and general malaise. These parameters are important to follow because improvements in these parameters often precede improvements in the physical findings and radiographic imaging associated with orbital cellulitis.

- Assess visual function. Visual acuity may be decreased, but is often unaffected by orbital cellulitis, although accurate measurement of acuity may be difficult to obtain, especially in pediatric patients. If an accurate measurement of acuity is not obtainable, additional assessments of visual function (eg, pupillary reaction, color vision) are critical not only for clinical and surgical decision making, but also for medical-legal documentation.

- The degree of globe displacement, extraocular motility limitation, as well as any retinal or optic nerve head findings should be documented.

- If trauma is suspected, the eyelids should be carefully examined for an entry wound of any potential foreign bodies.

- Radiographic imaging should be ordered whenever orbital cellulitis is suspected. Computed tomography scans provide excellent, rapid imaging of not only the orbital contents, but of the paranasal sinuses as well. Intravenous contrast should be used when possible because it may be useful in differentiating between a definite abscess formation in the orbit vs inflammatory phlegmatous involvement of orbital tissues. Magnetic resonance imaging also provides excellent imaging and may provide greater clarity in identifying the presence of an abscess or when intracranial extension is suspected.

Medical Therapy

- Although most cases of orbital cellulitis are caused by gram-positive organisms, particularly *Staphylococcus* and *Streptococcus* species, older patients or those with a history of chronic sinusitis may have polymicrobial infections. Therefore, it is still important to initiate broad-spectrum antibiotic coverage.[1]

- The most important step to successfully managing MRSA orbital cellulitis is to be aware of its level of activity in the hospital or community. This will allow you to initiate the appropriate antibiotic therapy. If your community has a low incidence of MRSA, then it may be appropriate to use nafcillin and cefotaxime to provide broad-spectrum coverage. Our region is associated with a very high incidence of community-acquired MRSA.[2] Therefore, at our institution, all patients presenting with orbital cellulitis are initially treated with vancomycin, cefotaxime, and either metronidazole or clindamycin. These antibiotics will then be changed according to patient response as well as the culture and antibiotic sensitivity results.

- Initiate aggressive nasal hygiene. A short course of a nasal decongestant such as oxymetazoline can facilitate drainage of the sinuses as well as an adjacent subperiosteal orbital abscess. Intranasal corticosteroids are also useful in decreasing nasal congestion, mucosal edema, and facilitating sinus drainage. Frequent use of saline nasal irrigations has been reported to facilitate sinus drainage as well.

- Consider the use of intravenous corticosteroids to control the inflammatory response associated with orbital cellulitis as well as facilitate the treatment of the associated sinusitis.[5] MRSA orbital abscesses have a tendency to be more loculated and have purulence of higher viscosity. The adjunct use of corticosteroids will often enhance the patient's response to medical therapy.

- Follow constitutional signs and visual function to assess the progress of medical therapy. Beware of worsening eyelid edema, proptosis, and increasing abscess size because the fluid load provided by the intravenous antibiotics can exacerbate these physical findings.

In most cases of orbital cellulitis, even those with MRSA, patients improve with medical therapy alone if the appropriate therapy is initiated. The first signs of improvement will be in the constitutional signs. Patients will defervesce and their overall sense of malaise will improve considerably. Surgery to drain a subperiosteal abscess should therefore be deferred unless there is worsening or lack of improvement with medical therapy, impending visual loss, or concurrent intracranial involvement.

Surgical Therapy

- After creating a transcutaneous, transcaruncular, or transconjunctival incision, blunt dissection is performed with scissors down to the periorbita adjacent to the subperiosteal abscess.[4]

- The orbital tissues are retracted and the periorbita is elevated posteriorly until the abscess is reached and the abscess contents are evacuated with suction. Using a suction trap, the abscess fluid can be collected and evaluated for culture and antibiotic sensitivities.

- A Penrose drain is placed into the abscess cavity and externalized through the surgical incision. This drain should be left in place for several days to monitor the amount of purulent drainage as well as to minimize the complications of postoperative orbital hemorrhage. If there is minimal drainage, the drain can be removed at the bedside.

Summary

Orbital cellulitis is a common condition with potentially devastating complications. Successful management of MRSA orbital cellulitis requires early identification of the infection and prompt initiation of the appropriate intravenous antibiotics. Surgical intervention may be necessary if the patient fails to respond to medical therapy, has impending visual loss, or if an associated foreign body is present in the orbit. Most cases of MRSA orbital cellulitis can be successfully treated. However, this may require close collaboration between the ophthalmologist, otolaryngologist, neurosurgeon, radiologist, pediatrician, microbiologist, and infectious disease consultant.

References

1. Garcia GH, Harris GJ. Criteria for nonsurgical management of subperiosteal abscess of the orbit: analysis of outcomes 1988-1998. *Ophthalmology*. 2000;107:1454-1456.

2. McKinley SH, Yen MT, Miller AM, Yen KG. Current trends in the microbiology of pediatric orbital cellulitis. *Am J Ophthalmol.* 2007;144:497-501.
3. Seltz LB, Smith J, Durairaj VD, Enzenauer R, Todd J. Microbiology and antibiotic management or orbital cellulitis. *Pediatrics.* 2011;127:e566-e572.
4. Pelton RW, Smith ME, Patel BCK, Kelly SM. Cosmetic considerations in surgery for orbital subperiosteal abscess in children: experience with a combined transcaruncular and transnasal endoscopic approach. *Arch Otolaryngol Head Neck Surg.* 2003;129:652-655.
5. Yen MT, Yen KG. The effect of corticosteroids in the acute management of pediatric orbital cellulitis with subperiosteal abscess. *Ophthal Plast Reconstr Surg.* 2005;21:363-366.

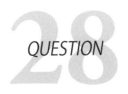

WHAT ARE THE GENERAL TREATMENT GUIDELINES FOR GRAVES' OPHTHALMOPATHY?

Jonathan W. Kim, MD

How often should I monitor my patients with Graves' disease? What are my nonsurgical options for managing exposure keratopathy? How long should they be stable before considering surgery? When is orbital decompression indicated and what technique do you recommend?

Graves' disease is the most common inflammatory process involving the orbits and adnexa. Although there are some variations in preferred terminology, when the eye disease occurs in conjunction with hyperthyroidism or the presence of thyroid-stimulating antibodies (eg, TSI), I like to use the label Graves' orbitopathy (GO). When ophthalmic changes occur in the setting of hypothyroidism or euthyroidism, I use the term *thyroid eye disease*.

Optimal management of GO requires a coordinated approach, addressing the thyroid dysfunction and ophthalmopathy. Progression can be influenced by certain lifestyle and systemic factors such as cigarette smoking, thyroid dysfunction, and radioactive iodine treatment for hyperthyroidism. Smoking increases the likelihood of progression of GO and retrospective evidence suggests that cessation of smoking improves the prognosis of the eye disease. The choice of antithyroid drug therapy or performance of thyroidectomy does not appear to affect the course of GO, but a minority of patients treated with radioactive iodine (15%) develop a worsening of the eye disease. Because this risk is greatly reduced by giving a short course of oral glucocorticoid therapy (0.3 to 0.5 mg/kg per day), prophylactic coverage should be considered in patients with moderate to severe GO.

Dating the onset of the ophthalmopathy is critical because the treatment algorithm is tailored to 1 of 3 stages of disease: (1) active-inflammatory, (2) stabilizing, and (3) quiescent. The NOSPECS classification system was used for many years to document the ophthalmic findings; my preference is for the more current VISA classification scheme (Table 28-1).[1] For ophthalmologists, the interval for monitoring is dependent on the clinical status of the patient; for patients

Kersten RC, McCulley TJ, eds. *Curbside Consultation in Oculoplastics: 49 Clinical Questions, Second Edition* (pp 137-141).
© 2016 Taylor & Francis Group.

Table 28-1

Summary of VISA Classification System for Graves' Ophthalmopathy

Vision		
Subjective	**Objective**	**OD/OS**
Vision (nl/abnl)	Central visual acuity	20/?
Color vision (nl/abnl)	Color vision errors Pupil abnormality (APD) Optic nerve edema Optic nerve pallor	Y/N
Inflammatory		
Subjective	**Objective**	
Retrobulbar ache (0 to 1)	Chemosis (0 to 2)	
Lid swelling (Y/N)	Conjunctival injection (0 to 1) Lid injection (0 to 1) Lid edema (0 to 2)	
Strabismus/Motility		
Subjective	**Objective**	
Diplopia (0 to 3)	Ductions (degrees)	
Head turn (Y/N)	Restriction (<15 to >45)	
Appearance/Exposure		
Subjective	**Objective**	
Lid retraction (Y/N)	Lid retraction (MRD)	
Proptosis (Y/N)	Levator function (mm)	
Tearing	Lagophthalmos (mm)	
Foreign body sensations (Y/N)	Exophthalmometry (Hertel) Corneal erosions/ulcerations Y/N IOP (upgaze, straight) mm Hg	
Grading		
V	Optic neuropathy	Y/N
I	Inflammation (0 to 8)	N/8
S	Strabismus (0 to 3) Restriction (0 to 3)	N/3 N/3
A	Appearance/exposure	Mild/moderate/severe

OD = right eye; OS = left eye; nl = normal; abnl = abnormal; APD = afferent pupillary defect; MRD = marginal reflex distance; IOP = intraocular pressure

Table 28-2

Clinical Evaluation of Graves' Ophthalmopathy

Exam Components	Initial Consultation	Follow-up Exam	Optic Neuropathy
Visual acuity	X	X	X
Color vision	X	X	X
Pupils	X	X	X
Motility	X	X	X
External exam (fissure height, lid lag)	X	X	X
Hertel exophthalmometry	X	X	X
Slit-lamp examination	X	X	X
IOP measurement	X	X	X
Dilated fundus exam	X	X*	X
Automated perimetry	X*		X
Diplopia fields (Goldmann perimeter)	X*	X*	

IOP = intraocular presurre
*Consider if clinically indicated.

with compressive optic neuropathy, assessments should be performed every 1 or 2 weeks, whereas patients who have active GO but no visual consequences can usually be seen every 6 to 8 weeks. I recommend evaluation of patients entering a stable phase every 3 to 4 months. Quiescent patients need only yearly follow-up exams. At every visit, GO patients should have a comprehensive ophthalmic evaluation (Table 28-2).

Fortunately, GO is mild and self-limited in the vast majority of patients and the natural history is one of slow improvement and stabilization. Symptoms of corneal exposure such as epiphora, photophobia, and foreign body sensation can be treated with frequent lubrication using preservative-free artificial tears. For recalcitrant cases, eyelid taping, moisture chambers, tarsorrhaphy, or botulinum toxin injections can be considered. Temporary lateral tarsorrhaphy and botulinum toxin injection (into levator muscle) should only be considered if there is a risk for corneal ulceration and permanent vision loss. For many patients in the inflammatory phase of GO, sleeping with the head elevated reduces the severity of periorbital edema and mechanical strabismus, particularly during the morning hours.

Recently, selenium has been recommended as a supplement for patients with mild, active GO to slow the progression of the eye disease. A randomized, double-blind, and placebo-controlled trial of 156 patients with mild GO compared the effects of selenium and pentoxifylline (anti-inflammatory) vs placebo.[2] A moderate dose of selenium (100 µg twice daily) given for 6 months was associated with improved quality of life, less eye involvement, and slower progression of

Figure 28-1. A 60-year-old patient with inflammatory Graves' orbitopathy, manifested by conjunctival injection (with hyperemia of the caruncle and restrictive strabismus), left optic neuropathy (20/50 vision), and only moderate proptosis.

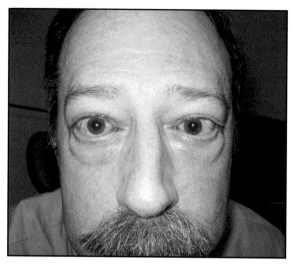

GO compared with placebo. The clinical activity score (CAS) also decreased in all groups, but the change was significantly greater in the selenium-treated patients. Subsequent evaluations at 12 months confirmed the results seen at 6 months. Selenium has antioxidative effects and it has been hypothesized that a reversal of the disturbed antioxidant balance in GO is responsible for this treatment effect, although the exact mechanisms have not been elucidated. As patients with Graves' disease begin to develop mild eye symptoms and signs, taking selenium as a supplement may be a safe way to moderate the severity of GO during its early stages.

Although the use of glucocorticoids in the management of patients with active, symptomatic GO is admittedly controversial, I have found them to be quite useful. In my opinion, they represent the most effective medical treatment for moderate to severe GO. For patients with severe inflammatory manifestations of GO, such as periorbital edema, congestive orbitopathy, and compressive optic neuropathy (Figure 28-1), systemic steroids are an effective temporizing measure, although the eye disease frequently recurs when the dose is tapered or withdrawn. Systemic steroids are not as effective for treating restrictive strabismus or extreme proptosis. For more on the use of immunosuppressive medications in the treatment of GO, see Question 22.

Orbital radiation is possibly more controversial as a treatment option for GO than the use of steroids. In the literature, there are very few randomized, prospective studies that support its routine use in Graves' patients. One randomized, controlled study demonstrated an improved outcome for GO patients with restrictive strabismus (vs sham treatment),[3] and there are numerous retrospective studies that suggest a therapeutic benefit for orbital radiotherapy in patients with compressive optic neuropathy. A contradictory, prospective, randomized, double-blind trial examining the effects of radiotherapy in GO found no difference in clinical outcomes between treated and untreated patients.[4] In clinical practice, orbital radiotherapy is mainly considered for patients in the inflammatory phase with progressive diplopia due to severe restrictive strabismus. Some clinicians also treat patients with severe inflammatory or congestive symptoms who have been on systemic steroids for longer than 3 months. This is discussed in more detail in Question 23.

Ideally, surgical management of GO patients proceeds in a fairly self-evident sequence: (1) orbital decompression, followed by (2) extraocular muscle surgery (strabismus repair), and finally (3) eyelid repositioning.[5] I like to defer soft tissue redraping (ie, blepharoplasty) until the 3 steps of functional reconstruction have been completed. When possible, rehabilitative surgery is reserved until patients have been documented to have inactive GO (with stable parameters) for at least 6 months. There are surgeons who like to wait for more than a year of stability. By waiting for quiescence, one can avoid reoperation for progressive disease and also any risk of causing a flare-up of the orbital inflammation. This, of course, only applies to the ideal situation; often medical necessity dictates that surgery be performed prior to a prolonged period of quiescence. For example, exposure keratopathy that has failed more conservative management options may require eyelid repositioning to be performed prior to stabilization. Similarly, a compressive optic neuropathy may require that orbital decompression be performed in the inflammatory phase of the disease.

Orbital decompression techniques have evolved significantly over the past 20 years. Traditionally, orbital decompression was associated with a 30% to 40% risk for consecutive strabismus. With modern techniques, the risk for consecutive diplopia is only 5% to 10% and more severe complications such as globe dystopia (eg, sun-setting syndrome) are rarely seen. This is, in part, due to the adoption of a balanced decompression, where the medial and lateral walls are taken, allowing for the floor to be left intact. Displacement of both the medial and lateral rectus muscles balances each, with less net globe deviation. Also, any misalignment is more apt to be in the horizontal plane, which is better compensated for because horizontal fusional amplitudes are much greater than vertical. Floor decompression is not able to be balanced with a roof decompression and any resulting vertical misalignment is more apt to manifest as a tropia. Other technical advances include strategic bone removal from the posterior orbit, removal of orbital fat, and use of smaller, hidden incisions. The inferomedial orbit and the posterior aspect of the orbital strut can be accessed endoscopically or through the conjunctival caruncle without creating a skin incision.[6] The deep lateral wall (diploic space of greater sphenoid wing) can be decompressed through an upper eyelid crease or lateral canthal incision. Orbital fat from the intraconal compartment can be debulked to provide a decompressive effect, either alone or in combination with bony removal. With improved surgical outcomes and decreased rates of complications, I often offer orbital decompression to GO patients with disfiguring proptosis and no visual symptoms.

Summary

As we gain better understanding of the pathophysiology of GO, management options will likely focus more on immune modulation. For the time being, surgery remains our therapeutic mainstay. Recent advancements in orbital decompression and eyelid repositioning allow for reconstruction to be performed more effectively and safely.

References

1. Dolman PJ, Rootman J. VISA classification for Graves' orbitopathy. *Ophthal Plast Reconstr Surg.* 2006;22(5):319-324.
2. Marcocci C, Kahaly GJ, Krassas GE, et al. Selenium and the course of mild Graves' orbitopathy. *N Engl J Med.* 2011;364(20):1920-1931.
3. Prummel MF, Terwee CB, Gerding MN, et al. A randomized controlled trial of orbital radiotherapy versus sham irradiation in patients with mild Graves' ophthalmopathy. *J Clin Endocrinol Metab.* 2004;89(1):13-14.
4. Gorman CA, Garrity JA, Fatourechi V, et al. A prospective, randomized, double-blind, placebo-controlled study of orbital radiotherapy for Graves' ophthalmopathy. *Ophthalmology.* 2001;108:1523-1534.
5. Shorr N, Seiff SR. The four stages of surgical rehabilitation of the patient with dysthyroid ophthalmopathy. *Ophthalmology.* 1986;93(4):476-483.
6. Kim JW, Goldberg RA, Shorr N. The inferomedial orbital strut: an anatomic and radiographic study. *Ophthal Plast Reconstr Surg.* 2002;18(5):355-564.

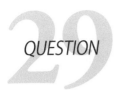

WHEN SHOULD CORTICOSTEROIDS BE USED FOR THYROID EYE DISEASE?

Mark J. Lucarelli, MD, FACS

Are there any published data comparing oral to intravenous steroid therapy? Are there any other immune modulators worth considering?

Although there are varying opinions among experts, corticosteroids are widely regarded as useful in the management of thyroid eye disease (TED). Several randomized, controlled trials have shown the value of oral corticosteroids in combination with low-dose orbital irradiation in treating severe inflammatory cases of thyroid orbitopathy. More recent trials have shown superiority of pulsed intravenous (IV) corticosteroids over oral steroid regimens in patients in the active inflammatory stage of the disease. Additionally, modest doses of oral corticosteroids have been proven useful as prophylactic treatment of patients with active thyroid eye disease who are about to undergo radioactive iodine ablation of the thyroid gland.

After reviewing the patient's history of endocrine dysfunction, it is important to obtain a careful history of the patient's ophthalmic manifestations of TED. It is important to try to establish the date when eye findings first were apparent. This can help establish how far the patient is along the course of the disease (Rundle's curve). Visual symptoms such as decreased acuity, decreased color vision, and visual field changes are critical because they can help point to a diagnosis of compressive or dysthyroid optic neuropathy (DON). Also, the presence of diplopia typically indicates restrictive myopathy. Worsening diplopia is generally indicative of disease progression. Ocular surface symptoms such as dryness, irritation, photophobia, and foreign body sensation are common but typically do not dictate treatment with systemic corticosteroids. It is important to ask about pain with eye movement, orbital pain at rest, redness of the eyes or the periocular skin, and swelling of the lids and conjunctiva—all of which may be indicative of active inflammation. Cigarette smoking should also be ascertained because it is a well-established and potent risk factor for worsening of TED.

Kersten RC, McCulley TJ, eds. *Curbside Consultation in Oculoplastics:*
49 Clinical Questions, Second Edition (pp 143-145).
© 2016 Taylor & Francis Group.

During the complete ophthalmic examination, it is important to look carefully for signs of active periocular and ocular inflammation. The presence of eyelid erythema and edema, conjunctival injection, and chemosis are often reliable signs of active periorbital inflammation. With the history and the exam findings, one can assign the patient a clinical activity score (CAS)[1] or a VISA-ITEDS[2] score.

Radioactive Iodine Ablation and Corticosteroids

An important randomized clinical trial has shown that some degree of worsening of TED occurs in about 15% of patients after radioactive iodine ablation (RAI).[3] In about two-thirds of patients who worsened, the change was transient. However, the other one-third had long-term, albeit mild, worsening of their thyroid eye disease. With the addition of prednisone (0.4 to 0.5 mg/kg per day) orally for 1 month and then tapered over the next 2 months for patients with CAS >3, this worsening of TED following RAI was completely prevented. A more recent study[4] has shown that reduced oral doses of 0.2 mg/kg prednisone tapered over 6 weeks have a similar protective effect.

In my practice, I generally recommend the following:

- If the patient has no signs of TED and is a nonsmoker, he or she could reasonably proceed with RAI without steroid prophylaxis.

- If the patient has any symptoms and signs of active, inflammatory TED, such as orbital pain at rest or with eye movement, eyelid erythema or edema, conjunctival chemosis or injection, I recommend prophylaxis with oral prednisone according to the reduced dosing (0.2 mg/kg) tapered over 1 month to 6 weeks.

- It is essential to urge smokers to cease smoking, especially if RAI is being considered.

- It is worthwhile to remind the patient's endocrinologist that maintaining a euthyroid state is desirable for the eyes. Postablation hypothyroidism[5] is an accepted risk factor for ophthalmopathy.

Corticosteroids for Active Thyroid Eye Disease or Dysthyroid Optic Neuropathy

The literature provides less dependable guidance on when to (or whether to) initiate corticosteroids in the setting of active (inflammatory) thyroid eye disease. As such, one must try to balance the risk for systemic steroid-related morbidity with the anticipated benefit of steroid treatment. The difficulty of predicting the duration and the eventual severity of the thyroid orbitopathy makes clinical decision making in this area even more challenging.

In moderately severe to severe active thyroid orbitopathy, high-dose glucocorticoids are generally considered first-line treatment. Recent literature has shown increased efficacy and decreased morbidity with pulsed IV corticosteroids as compared with oral corticosteroids. A prospective single-blind trial[6] by Marcocci et al showed favorable results in 88% of patients receiving pulsed IV corticosteroids and radiotherapy compared with 63% for those receiving oral treatment and radiotherapy.

A randomized clinical trial[7] by Kahaly et al compared oral vs IV corticosteroid therapy in the setting of active thyroid eye disease. The IV regimen consisted of once weekly steroid infusions (0.5 gm methylprednisolone × 6 weeks, followed by 250 mg weekly for 6 weeks, for a total dose of 4.5 gm methylprednisolone). A treatment response was noted in 77% of patients treated with the IV regimen compared with 51% for patients treated with oral corticosteroids. Additionally, significantly fewer patients in the IV group sustained steroid-related complications. Work published by Bartalena et al on behalf of the European Group of Graves' Orbitopathy has also shown similar results.[8]

In the setting of severe, active thyroid eye disease, pulsed IV corticosteroid therapy offers advantages over oral regimens. I recommend the protocol described by Kahaly (500 mg methylprednisolone infusion weekly × 6 weeks, followed by 250 mg weekly × 6 weeks). Careful systemic monitoring (including assessment of risk for liver toxicity and monitoring hepatic function) is performed by the patient's internist or endocrinologist. Courses of high-dose oral corticosteroids, especially beyond 8 to 12 weeks, or without some specific planned endpoint, are particularly avoided given the high incidence of morbidity. Smoking cessation is urged, as in any patient with thyroid eye disease.

For patients with thyroid optic neuropathy, high-dose oral corticosteroids at about 80 mg prednisone orally × 5 days can be initiated until the Kahaly pulsed IV therapy can be arranged. Visual function is monitored closely. In severe cases of optic neuropathy, a low threshold for surgical decompression is maintained. If significant improvement is not noted in severe cases in about 1 to 2 weeks, prompt surgical orbital decompression is usually carried out. In less severe cases of thyroid optic neuropathy, consideration is given to low-dose orbital irradiation (2000 cGy in 10 divided fractions over 2 weeks) if treatment with steroids produces an incomplete or transient therapeutic response.

Beyond Corticosteroids

In patients with severe inflammatory TED with contraindications to pulsed IV corticosteroids, consideration can be given for use of rituximab. This agent results in temporary depletion of CD-20+ B-cells. After initial publication by Salvi et al, several reports have shown efficacy of rituximab in this setting.[9,10] The risk for the highly feared complication of progressive multifocal leukoencephalopathy is felt to be very modest at about 1/25000. Randomized clinical trials attempting to clarify the role and optimal dosing of rituximab in severe inflammatory TED are underway.

References

1. Mourits MP, Koornneef L, Wiersinga WM, et al. Clinical criteria for the assessment of disease activity in Graves' ophthalmopathy: a novel approach. *Br J Ophthalmol.* 1989;73(8):639-644.
2. Dolman PJ, Rootman J. VISA classification for Graves' orbitopathy. *Ophthal Plast Reconstr Surg.* 2006;22:319-324.
3. Bartalena L, Marcocci C, Bogazzi F, et al. Relation between therapy for hyperthyroidism and the course of Graves' ophthalmopathy. *N Eng J Med.* 1998;338:73-78.
4. Lai A, Sassi L, Compri E, et al. Lower dose prednisone prevents radioiodine-associated exacerbation of initially mild or absent Graves' orbitopathy. *J Clin Endocrinol Metab.* 2010;95:1333-1337.
5. Perros P, Kendall-Taylor P, Neoh C, et al. A prospective study of the effects of radioiodine therapy for hyperthyroidism in patients with minimally active Graves' ophthalmopathy. *J Clin Endocrinol Metab.* 2005;90:5321-5323.
6. Marcocci C, Bartalena L, Tanda ML, et al. Comparison of the effectiveness and tolerability of intravenous or oral glucocorticoids associated with orbital radiotherapy in the management of severe Graves' ophthalmopathy. *J Clin Endocrinol Metab.* 2001;86:3562-3567.
7. Kahaly GJ, Pitz S, Hommel G, Dittmar M. Randomized, single blind trial of intravenous versus oral steroid monotherapy in patients with Graves' orbitopathy. *J Clin Endocrinol Metab.* 2005;90:5234-5240.
8. Bartalena L, Krassas GE, Wiersinga W, et al. Efficacy and safety of three different cumulative doses of intravenous methylprednisolone for moderate to severe and active Graves' orbitopathy. *J Clin Endocrinol Metab.* 2012;97:4454-4563.
9. Silkiss RZ, Reier A, Coleman M, Lauer SA. Rituximab for thyroid eye disease. *Ophth Plast Reconstr Surg.* 2010;26:310-314.
10. Salvi M, Vannucchi G, Curro N, et al. Small dose rituximab for Graves' orbitopathy. *Arch Ophthalmol.* 2012;130:122-124.

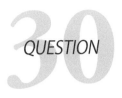

QUESTION

Do You Think Radiation Is Ever Indicated for Graves' Disease?

Vikram D. Durairaj, MD

Didn't the Mayo study demonstrate that radiation has no effect in Graves' patients? Is there a subgroup of patients that it should be reserved for?

The role of orbital radiation to treat orbital inflammatory signs and compressive optic neuropathy associated with thyroid eye disease is widely debated. Let us briefly review what the literature tells us.

Gorman et al conducted a prospective, randomized, double-masked, placebo-controlled clinical trial (The Mayo Orbital Radiotherapy for Graves' Ophthalmopathy Study) to examine the clinical benefit of orbital radiation in patients with mild to moderate thyroid eye disease.[1] The authors studied 42 consecutive patients with moderate, symptomatic Graves' ophthalmopathy (GO). One orbit was randomized to treatment with 20 Gy of external beam therapy and the other orbit was treated with sham therapy. The treatments were reversed 6 months later. They concluded that when assessed at 1 year after initiating treatment, radiotherapy had been ineffective in managing patients with mild to moderate GO.[1] The authors in a 3-year uncontrolled follow-up of the same patients confirmed that orbital radiotherapy is not indicated for the treatment of mild to moderate GO.[2] It should be noted that patients with compressive optic neuropathy were not included in this study. Critics of the Mayo study state that the group of patients examined did not represent the types of patients that can most benefit from orbital radiotherapy. These include patients with optic neuropathy, steroid-dependent orbital inflammation, and rapidly progressing orbitopathy. I believe that it is safe to conclude from the Mayo study that orbital radiotherapy is not effective for patients in the stable phase of GO. However, I think that it would be inappropriate to conclude that radiation therapy has no role in the management of Graves' patients.

There are numerous studies that have supported the use of orbital radiotherapy in the treatment of GO. Two randomized, controlled studies by Mourits et al and Prummel et al demonstrated

147

Kersten RC, McCulley TJ, eds. Curbside Consultation in Oculoplastics:
49 Clinical Questions, Second Edition (pp 147-149).
© 2016 Taylor & Francis Group.

that orbital radiotherapy is more effective than sham irradiation in improving diplopia and eye muscle motility.[3,4] The consensus statement of the European Group on Graves' Orbitopathy on Management of Graves' Orbitopathy states that orbital irradiation should be considered in patients with active disease who have diplopia or restrictive myopathy.[5] Kazim has also presented data in support of the effectiveness of orbital radiotherapy in the treatment of patients with compressive optic neuropathy.[6] Bradley et al have nicely summarized the evidence-based role of orbital radiation in the treatment of thyroid eye disease.[7]

Let us review some important details concerning orbital radiotherapy for the treatment of GO. Various treatment regimens have been proposed. Recent trends have been toward lower total doses of radiation, spread out over a greater period. Traditionally, treatment involved a cumulative dose of 20 Gy per orbit fractionated in 10 doses over a 2-week period. Recently, less aggressive regimens have been gaining popularity—a lower dose of 10 Gy or an alternative treatment regimen of 1 Gy per week over a 20-week period. These "lesser" regimens may prove equally effective and better tolerated than the standard regimen. Another consideration is combining corticosteroids with radiation. This may prove more effective than orbital radiation alone.

Complications of orbital radiotherapy include cataract formation, retinal microvascular abnormalities, and the theoretical risk for carcinogenesis in younger patients. Due to an increased risk for vascular damage, orbital radiation is often avoided in patients with diabetes and severe hypertension. However, complications from orbital radiotherapy are not common and, in my opinion, do not outweigh the benefits in properly selected patients.

My personal approach and incorporation of radiation therapy agrees with the Mayo Study—not all patients with Graves' will benefit from radiation therapy. I generally perform surgical decompression on patients with compressive optic neuropathy, in part because the benefits of radiation are often delayed and rapid decompression is more apt to salvage lost vision. However, I will recommend radiation to patients with continued compression of their optic nerves, despite having been maximally decompressed. I will sometimes use radiation therapy as a first-line therapy in patients who have medical conditions, making them poor surgical candidates. In general, patients with active inflammation will respond better than those with more mature, burnt out disease. I also think it is reasonable to treat these patients with radiation in combination with corticosteroids. Finally, I also believe patients with rapidly progressing or steroid-dependent orbitopathy can be treated successfully with orbital radiation.

Summary

I believe that orbital radiotherapy is effective and safe in patients with active thyroid eye disease. Although I prefer surgical decompression for patients with compressive optic neuropathy, radiotherapy can be offered to patients in active phase of disease. It is most effective in combination with glucocorticoids and may improve thyroid eye disease associated optic neuropathy, dysmotility, and inflammatory periocular.[8] A large, prospective, randomized trial is needed before stating with certainty the best treatment options.

References

1. Gorman CA, Garrity JA, Fatourechi V, et al. A prospective, randomized, double-blind, placebo-controlled study of orbital radiotherapy for Graves' ophthalmopathy. *Ophthalmology.* 2001;108:1523-1534.
2. Gorman CA, Garrity JA, Fatourechi V, et al. The aftermath of orbital radiotherapy for Graves' ophthalmopathy. *Ophthalmology.* 2002;109(11):2100-2107.
3. Mourits MP, van Kempen-Harteveld ML, García MB, Koppeschaar HP, Tick L, Terwee CB. Radiotherapy for Graves' orbitopathy: randomised placebo-controlled study. *Lancet.* 2000;355:1505-1509.

4. Prummel MF, Terwee CB, Gerding MN, et al. A randomized controlled trial of orbital radiotherapy versus sham irradiation in patients with mild Graves' ophthalmopathy. *J Clin Endocrinol Metab*. 2004;89:15-20.

5. Bartalena L, Baldeschi L, Dickinson AJ, et al. Consensus statement of the European group on Graves' orbitopathy on management of Graves' orbitopathy. *Thyroid*. 2008;18(3):333-346.

6. Kazim M. Perspective—Part II: radiotherapy for Graves' orbitopathy: the Columbia University experience. *Ophthal Plast Reconstr Surg*. 2002;18:173-174.

7. Bradley EA, Gower EW, Bradley DJ, et al. Orbital radiation for Graves' ophthalmopathy: a report by the American Academy of Ophthalmology. *Ophthalmology*. 2008:115(2):398-409.

8. Dolman PJ, Rath S. Orbital radiotherapy for thyroid eye disease. *Curr Opin Ophthal*. 2012;23(5):427-432.

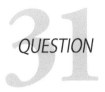

SHOULD LOCAL CHEMOTHERAPY PLAY A ROLE IN THE MANAGEMENT OF LACRIMAL OR OTHER ORBITAL MALIGNANCY?

Andrea Lora Kossler, MD

I recently saw a patient with an adenoid cystic carcinoma of the lacrimal gland. He had received conflicting recommendations about treatment. What are your thoughts on local chemotherapy, with or without surgery?

Lacrimal Gland Malignancy and Treatment Options

Adenoid cystic carcinoma (ACC) of the lacrimal gland accounts for 1.6% of all orbital tumors and is well known for its aggressive biological behavior, with a proclivity for perineural and bony infiltration. Local recurrence, distant metastasis, and retrograde intracranial extension via the lacrimal nerve are common.

A study by Font and Gamel[1] reported a dismal actuarial survival rate of about 20% at 10 years regardless of therapy, which included globe sparing local excision, exenteration, radiation, exenteration combined with radiation (RT), and an unspecified chemotherapeutic protocol. The poor prognosis with current treatment options is due to the inability to address occult metastases even after surgery and radiation therapy has achieved local disease control. Currently, the optimal management for ACC is a subject of great controversy with a paucity of long-term data available to guide therapy.

Intra-arterial Cytoreductive Chemotherapy for Lacrimal Gland Malignancy

Intra-arterial infusion has been used for the treatment of central nervous system tumors, primary and metastatic liver tumors, and select breast tumors. Meldrum et al[2] introduced the

Kersten RC, McCulley TJ, eds. *Curbside Consultation in Oculoplastics:*
49 Clinical Questions, Second Edition (pp 151-161).
© 2016 Taylor & Francis Group.

neoadjuvant intra-arterial cytoreductive chemotherapy (IACC) protocol for lacrimal gland malignancy treatment in 1998. The rationale of chemotherapy treatment was to administer a high concentration of a chemotherapeutic agent to the lacrimal gland tumor through the anastomotic branches of the external carotid artery (ECA) vascular system, prior to surgical excision of the tumor, to enhance tumor cell death and shrink tumor size. Additionally, IACC can minimize viable tumor cell dissemination during surgical manipulation and introduces systemic therapy early in the course of treatment to address micrometastatic disease and achieve improved locoregional control. The advantage of the ECA intra-arterial (IA) route is that its concentration is considerably higher than that with intravenous (IV) delivery while avoiding direct brain perfusion.

The IACC protocol is completed through a multidisciplinary team approach comprised of an experienced medical oncologist, an interventional radiologist, and an oculoplastic surgeon. The protocol begins with 2 cycles of IA drug infusion at 3-week intervals. Cisplatin (100 mg/m^2) is delivered via a catheter inserted through the ipsilateral femoral artery to the ECA under angiographic control. The dose of cisplatin is diluted in 500 mL of normal saline solution and delivered over 1 hour. Immediately following the cisplatin infusion, the catheter is removed and doxorubicin hydrochloride (25 mg/m^2 per day) is given intravenously. Additional doxorubicin hydrochloride (25 mg/m^2 per day) is given on 2 subsequent days. The patient is hospitalized during the 3 days of treatment and hydrated with 250 mL D5 0.45% NS to achieve a urine output greater than 150 mL per hour. Antiemetic premedication consists of odansteron hydrochloride, dexamethasone sodium phosphate, and lorazepam. The patient is monitored for neutropenia, fever, and catheter-related complications. Following hematologic recovery, orbital imaging is done to assess tumor response. A third cycle may be given if further tumor shrinkage would allow complete resection with exenteration. Three to 4 weeks later, orbital exenteration is performed. About 6 weeks after surgery, standard daily fractional radiation therapy (55 to 60 Gy) is delivered in combination with IV radiosensitizing cisplatin (20 mg/m^2) once weekly on an outpatient basis. Four weeks after radiation therapy, the patient is retreated with 4 cycles of IV cisplatin (100 mg/m^2) and doxorubicin (20 mg/m^2) daily for 3 days. This protocol results in a total of 6 cycles of systemic therapy—2 IA and 4 IV.

Risk factors for suboptimal response to IACC include (1) extent of disease or breach of orbital boundaries at presentation; (2) failure to obtain a preoperative incisional biopsy prior to surgical planning; (3) surgical disruption of the lateral orbital wall, tumor manipulation, and incomplete tumor resection; (4) absence of an intact lacrimal artery to maximize drug delivery; and (5) failure to implement all parts of the IACC protocol. To begin treatment of any suspicious lacrimal gland malignancy, an initial transcutaneous incisional biopsy without bone removal is recommended to preserve the lacrimal artery and blood supply to the lacrimal gland. If there is concern for pleomorphic adenoma, cyanoacrylate glue can be used to cover the incisional biopsy site to minimize tumor cell spillage while waiting for intraoperative frozen tissue diagnosis. If the biopsy reveals ACC, the incision site is closed and the IACC protocol can begin. This will avoid extensive surgical disruption of the bone and tumor bed, which will compromise the blood supply to the lacrimal gland and interfere with IACC drug delivery through the lacrimal artery. Finally, once the protocol begins, it is critical to complete all elements of the protocol in a timely manner to completely eradicate tumor cells and avoid interval tumor regrowth.

Intra-arterial Cytoreductive Chemotherapy for Lacrimal Gland Adenoid Cystic Carcinoma

In 2013, Tse et al[3] reported the long-term follow-up of 21 patients, enrolled over 24 years, treated with the IACC protocol for lacrimal gland malignancy. Nineteen of these patients were treated for ACC while 2 were treated for adenocarcinoma (Table 31-1). The patients treated for ACC were separated into 2 groups: Group 1 was composed of 8 patients with an intact lacrimal artery who completed the IACC treatment protocol and Group 2 included 11 patients who deviated from the protocol design or presented without an intact lacrimal artery. During a median follow-up of 10 years (range 2 to 24 years), survival in Group 1 patients was a remarkable 100%, with all 8 patients remaining disease free. The cumulative survival at 10 years in Group 2 was 72%. Both groups fared far better than any previous long-term reports.

Safety and Toxicity of Local Chemotherapy

Tse et al[3] report that out of 51 IACC procedures, the treatment was safe and well tolerated by most patients. There were 5 episodes of febrile neutropenia (5/51 or 9.8%) after IA infusion. Additionally, 9 patients experienced trismus, 6 experienced ototoxicity, and 2 had transient facial paresis. The side effects to treatment were manageable by trained medical oncologists. There were no catheter-related and/or angiographic complications such as thrombotic stroke, hemorrhage, or ophthalmologic toxicity when chemotherapy was delivered through the ECA. There was one case of internal carotid artery infusion that resulted in vessel thrombosis, no light perception vision, anterior segment ischemia, and forehead hyperpigmentation (Figure 31-1). This case supports the ECA route to avoid ocular complication and brain toxicity.

Summary

Lacrimal gland malignancies evoke a dismal prognosis with conventional treatments. The introduction of intra-arterial chemotherapy infusion has resulted in remarkable improvement in disease-free survival and local control rates. Long-term survival findings affirm that this approach is an appropriate local chemotherapeutic technique for effective disease treatment and that local chemotherapy treatment is well tolerated by most patients. The IACC protocol should be considered for any patient with non-lymphoid lacrimal gland malignancy and should be implemented by an experienced multidisciplinary team.

Table 31-1

Patient Characteristics of IA Cytoreductive Chemotherapy and Conventional Treatment for Adenoid Cystic Carcinoma of the Lacrimal Gland

Patient No.	Age/ Gender/ Affected Side	ACC Subtype/ Perineural/ Bone Infiltration	IACC Cycles/ Total Cycles	Prior Tumor Resection	Radiographic Tumor Response/ Tissue Margins	Treatment	Time (mo) of and Status at Last Follow-up	Time (mo) of Local Recurrence/ Met	Remarks
Group 1									
1	29/M/OD	Basa/P/B	3/4	No	Yes/–	Exent + RT	288; Alive, no D	No	Intracranial
3	73/F/OS	Basa/P	2/6	No	Yes/–	Exent + RT	193; Alive, no D	No	Kidney transplant
4	58/M/OS	Crib	2/6	No	Yes/–	Exent + RT + GK	156; Alive, no D	No	Intracranial,
5	35/M/OS	Crib/P	3/6	No	Yes/+	Exent + RT	149, Alive, no D	No	Non-healing apex; free flap
7	30/M/OS	Basa/P	2/4	No	Yes/–	Exent + Bone + RT	116; Alive, no D	No	
10	29/F/OD	Basa	2/6	No	Yes/–	Exent + RT	96; Alive; no D	No	

(continued)

Table 31-1 (continued)

Patient Characteristics of IA Cytoreductive Chemotherapy and Conventional Treatment for Adenoid Cystic Carcinoma of the Lacrimal Gland

Patient No.	Age/ Gender/ Affected Side	ACC Subtype/ Perineural/ Bone Infiltration	IACC Cycles/ Total Cycles	Prior Tumor Resection	Radiographic Tumor Response/ Tissue Margins	Treatment	Time (mo) of and Status at Last Follow-up	Time (mo) of Local Recurrence/ Met	Remarks
Group 1									
17	53/F/OD	Basa	2/6	No	Yes/–	Exent + RT	29; Alive; no D	No	Neck dissection negative
18	44/M/OS	Basa/Crib/ P/B	3/6	No	Yes/+	Exent + RT	20; Alive; no D	No	Lung Bx negative
Group 2									
2	32/M/OD	Crib/P/B	3/6	Yes	Yes/–	Exent + Bone + RT	167; Died; no D	No	HIV, died of oral SCC
6	42/F/OD	Crib/P/B	3/6	Yes	Yes/–	Exent + Bone + RT	127; Alive; with D	50; Lung	Bone necrosis, hearing deficint; 7th N palsy

(continued)

Table 31-1 (continued)

Patient Characteristics of IA Cytoreductive Chemotherapy and Conventional Treatment for Adenoid Cystic Carcinoma of the Lacrimal Gland

Patient No.	Age/ Gender/ Affected Side	ACC Subtype/ Perineural/ Bone Infiltration	IACC Cycles/ Total Cycles	Prior Tumor Resection	Radiographic Tumor Response/ Tissue Margins	Treatment	Time (mo) of and Status at Last Follow-up	Time (mo) of Local Recurrence/ Met	Remarks
Group 2									
8	36/F/OS	Basa/P/B	2/2	No	Yes/+	Exent + RT	28; Died of D	18; LR/Liver	Delayed exent, refused final 4 cycles
9	64/F/OD	Crib/B	2/2	Yes	Yes/+	Exent orbit/sinuses + Bone + RT	112; Alive; no D	13; LR/Sinus	Delayed exent, refused final 4 cycles, ACC in sinus mucosa resected

(continued)

Table 31-1 (continued)

Patient Characteristics of IA Cytoreductive Chemotherapy and Conventional Treatment for Adenoid Cystic Carcinoma of the Lacrimal Gland

Patient No.	Age/ Gender/ Affected Side	ACC Subtype/ Perineural/ Bone Infiltration	IACC Cycles/ Total Cycles	Prior Tumor Resection	Radiographic Tumor Response/ Tissue Margins	Treatment	Time (mo) of and Status at Last Follow-up	Time (mo) of Local Recurrence/ Met	Remarks
Group 2									
11	54/M/OS	Crib/Basa	2/6	Yes	Yes/+	Exent + Bone + TM + RT	87; Died of D	20; LR/ Lung/Brain	Extensive disease at presentation
12	32/F/OD	Crib	2/5	Yes	Yes/+	Exent + Bone + RT + GK	85; Alive; no D	No	
13	34/M/OD	Crib	2/6	Yes	Yes/–	Exent + Bone + RT	89; Alive; no D	No	Ophthal artery infusion, vessel thrombosis
14	49/M/OS	Crib/Basa	2/5	Yes	Yes/–	Exent + Bone + RT	82; Alive; no D	60; Lung	NED after lung nodule resection

(continued)

Table 31-1 (continued)

Patient Characteristics of IA Cytoreductive Chemotherapy and Conventional Treatment for Adenoid Cystic Carcinoma of the Lacrimal Gland

Patient No.	Age/ Gender/ Affected Side	ACC Subtype/ Perineural/ Bone Infiltration	IACC Cycles/ Total Cycles	Prior Tumor Resection	Radiographic Tumor Response/ Tissue Margins	Treatment	Time (mo) of and Status at Last Follow-up	Time (mo) of Local Recurrence/ Met	Remarks
Group 2									
15	20/M/OD	Crib/Basa/ P/B	3/5	Yes	Yes/–	Exent + Bone + RT	73; Alive; no D	No	
16	38/F/OS	Basa	2/6	Yes	Yes/+	Exent + RT	52; Alive; no D	No	
19	56/M/OS	Basa/P	5/5	Yes	Yes/+	Exent orbit/sinus-es + RT	20; Alive; no D	No	Intracranial; ACC in sinus mucosa, free flap

(continued)

Table 31-1 (continued)

Patient Characteristics of IA Cytoreductive Chemotherapy and Conventional Treatment for Adenoid Cystic Carcinoma of the Lacrimal Gland

Patient No.	Age/ Gender/ Affected Side	ACC Subtype/ Perineural/ Bone Infiltration	IACC Cycles/ Total Cycles	Prior Tumor Resection	Radiographic Tumor Response/ Tissue Margins	Treatment	Time (mo) of and Status at Last Follow-up	Time (mo) of Local Recurrence/ Met	Remarks
Alternate Histology									
20	43/F/OS	Adenocar/ P/B	2/6	Yes	Yes/–	Exent + RT	41; Died; no D	No	No ACC detected in exenteration specimen; AML 3 years post IACC; 11q23 translocation
21	45/F/OD	Adenocar/ P/B	2/2	No	Yes/+	Exent +RT	30; Died of D	26; Brain	+ margin at superior orbital fissure

(continued)

Table 31-1 (continued)

Patient Characteristics of IA Cytoreductive Chemotherapy and Conventional Treatment for Adenoid Cystic Carcinoma of the Lacrimal Gland

ACC = adenoid cystic carcinoma; Basa = basaloid subtype; Crib = cribiform subtype; B = bone infiltration; P = perineural infiltration; Radiographic Tumor Response/Tissue Margins = radiographic evidence of tumor shrinkage after IA chemotherapy cycles/presence of tumor cells at soft tissue surgical margins; No D = No ACC; LR = local recurrence; Met = distant metastases; D = disease (local or metastatic ACC); Exent + bone + RT = exenteration with removal of lateral orbital wall fragment plus postoperative radiation therapy; TM = temporalis muscle resection; Exent + RT = exenteration plus postoperative radiation therapy; GK = gamma knife therapy; NED = no evidence of disease; N/A = not applicable; Resect = primary resection of mass; SCC = squamous cell carcinoma; 7th N = facial nerve palsy; Adenocar = adenocarcinoma; AML = acute myelocytic leukemia.

Reprinted with permission from Tse DT, Kossler AL, Feuer WJ, Benedetto PW. Long-term outcomes of neoadjuvant intraarterial cytoreductive chemotherapy for lacrimal gland adenoid cystic carcinoma. *Ophthalmology.* 2013;120(7):1313-1323. © 2013 Elsevier.

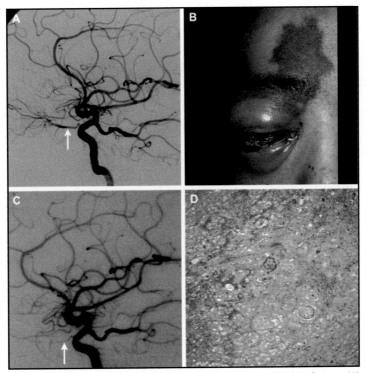

Figure 31-1. Complication of internal carotid artery (ICA) infusion. (A) Diagnostic ICA angiogram showing tumor remnants supplied by the ophthalmic artery (arrow). (B) Skin hyperpigmentation over the medial right brow and forehead. Anterior segment examination showing conjunctival injection, chemosis, hemorrhage, corneal edema, shallow anterior chamber, and hypotony. (C) Repeat angiogram showing a hypoplastic right ophthalmic artery (arrow). (D) Histopathologic examination of an exenterated specimen shows foci of tumor necrosis and blood vessel thrombosis. (Reprinted with permission from Tse DT, Kossler AL, Feuer WJ, Benedetto PW. Long-term outcomes of neoadjuvant intraarterial cytoreductive chemotherapy for lacrimal gland adenoid cystic carcinoma. *Ophthalmology.* 2013;120(7):1313-1323. © 2013 Elsevier.)

References

1. Font RL, Gamel JW. Adenoid cystic carcinoma of the lacrimal gland: a clinicopathologic study of 79 cases. In Nicholson DH, ed. *Ocular Pathology Update.* New York: Masson; 1980:277-283.
2. Meldrum ML, Tse DT, Benedetto P. Neoadjuvant intracarotid chemotherapy for treatment of advanced adenocystic carcinoma of the lacrimal gland. *Arch Ophthalmol.* 1998;116(3):315-321.
3. Tse DT, Kossler AL, Feuer WJ, Benedetto PW. Long-term outcomes of neoadjuvant intra-arterial cytoreductive chemotherapy for lacrimal gland adenoid cystic carcinoma. *Ophthalmology.* 2013;120(7):1313-1323.

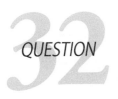

QUESTION

WHAT IS NEW IN THE
MANAGEMENT OF ORBITAL LYMPHOMA?

Timothy J. Sullivan, FRANZCO

What clues are there that orbital diseases are due to lymphoproliferative disease? What are the best diagnostic tests? Are there any new chemotherapeutic options?

There have been major advances in our understanding of the pathogenesis of Ocular Adnexal Lymphoproliferative disease (OALD) and some of its subtypes, refinements in imaging and staging, not to mention modifications to treatment that the general ophthalmologist needs to know.[1] The role of not just the cell type (eg, mantle vs marginal zone) but its microenvironment is of critical importance in patient response and outcome. We have seen recent advances in our understanding of orbital IgG4 inflammatory disease and its overlap with lymphoproliferative disease. You can read more about this in Question 26. Full understanding of the role of infectious agents remains elusive but is nonetheless germane. There have been advances in the use of positron emission tomography (PET) scanning for staging, response to treatment, and possible relapse. Diffusion-weighted imaging (DWI magnetic resonance imaging [MRI]) has also become a helpful tool not only in diagnosis but in assessing response to treatment. With distillations of the WHO classification and directed laboratory efforts, we also have a clearer picture of how the individual lymphoma entities such as marginal zone, follicular, mantle, and diffuse large B cell lymphomas behave in the ocular adnexal region.[2,3] All these factors and modifications of existing protocols have led to incremental progress in treatment.

Figure 32-1 illustrates a 65-year-old patient who presented with a painless conjunctival salmon patch in the superior fornix when the upper lid was manually elevated. This may be a typical presentation of lymphoma, but sometimes there can be atypical presentations with varying degrees of pain or inflammation, particularly in younger patients or those with more aggressive disease.

The most important role of the ophthalmologist is to consider the diagnosis of lymphoma for every orbital case, to arrange appropriate imaging studies (computed tomography [CT] or MRI of the brain, orbits, and sinuses) and to take a biopsy specimen that will confirm the diagnosis and allow correct subtyping. This requires an adequate tissue sample, taking care to avoid artifact

Kersten RC, McCulley TJ, eds. *Curbside Consultation in Oculoplastics: 49 Clinical Questions, Second Edition* (pp 163-166).
© 2016 Taylor & Francis Group.

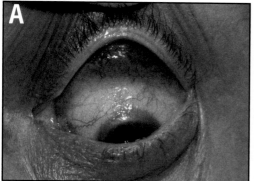
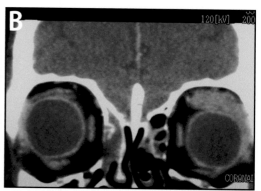
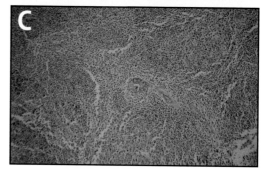

Figure 32-1. (A) Clinical photograph showing typical adnexal MALT lymphoma presenting as a salmon patch. (B) Coronal soft tissue winder CT scan of the patient seen in (A), showing a well-circumscribed mass in the superior aspect of the left orbit molding to the globe. (C) Low power (×100) histological (hemotoxylin-eosin) section of a typical MALT lymphoma showing centrocyte-like monocytoid cells, plasmacytoid cells, and follicular colonization, as well as a characteristic lymphoepithelial lesion (center).

due to crushing or diathermy. Fresh tissue taken at the time permits imprints and frozen section, which can give an early clue to diagnosis and ensure that representative tissue has been sampled. Fresh tissue should also be placed in lymphoma transport medium for flow cytometry, as well as formalin for paraffin sections and immunohistochemistry. Subsequently, abnormal nucleic acid or products produced by the DNA abnormality can be detected. This can be performed by most pathology laboratories with expertise in lymphoma using immunohistochemistry and molecular genetic studies such as polymerase chain reaction (PCR) and fluorescent in situ hybridization (FISH). Comparative genomic hybridization and gene expression profiling using cDNA microarray technology are research tools but will increasingly be integrated into diagnostic testing.

These techniques should allow the majority of OALDs to be diagnosed as malignant lymphoma (usually 80% to 90%) or a reactive lymphoid hyperplasia (RLH 10% to 20%). Occasionally, this distinction cannot be made, resulting in an intermediate diagnosis of atypical lymphoid hyperplasia (<5%). Here, the overlap with IgG4-related orbital disease (IgG4 ROD) is important. Many lesions previously described as pseudotumor, idiopathic orbital inflammation, and reactive lymphoid hyperplasia are in fact due to IgG4 ROD. Further, some truly monoclonal orbital lymphomas have been shown to arise from IgG4 ROD.[4] OALD is classified using the WHO modification of the revised European-American Lymphoma classification. OALD are all extranodal and the majority are classified as marginal zone B-cell lymphomas. These are low-grade lymphomas that are identical to mucosa associated lymphoid tumors (MALT), occurring most commonly in the gastrointestinal tract. They are associated with mucosa in the conjunctiva, but not in the orbit and eyelid. Some prefer that the term *MALT* be limited to those lesions arising in the gastrointestinal tract and that similar lesions in the orbit be referred to simply as marginal zone B-cell lymphomas. This distinction makes sense because lesions in the 2 areas have different cytogenetic profiles. Most large series confirm the extranodal marginal zone lymphoma to comprise between 50% to 70% of OALD. Other common indolent lesions include follicular and lymphoplasmacytic lymphoma, while the 2 more common aggressive lesions are the diffuse large B-cell lymphoma

(DLBCL) and Mantle lymphoma (MCL). Rarely, other non-Hodgkin B-cell lesions (eg, small cell lymphoma) may occur and T-cell lymphomas also occur rarely.

Once a diagnosis has been established, management should be multidisciplinary including the ophthalmologist, hematologist, and radiation oncologist. A full medical history should be taken, with clinical examination including palpation of lymph nodes, liver, and spleen. Staging of OALD has been revolutionized by the application of the American Joint Committee on Cancer TNM staging system for OALD. This was introduced to overcome shortcomings in the Ann Arbor system for OALD and to allow more accurate staging that could correlate better with treatment and outcomes.

Initial tests including complete blood counts with cytologic examination, LDH and beta-2-microglobulin levels, evaluation of renal and hepatic function, serology for hepatitis C virus (HCV), and HIV infections. Bone marrow analysis is mandatory. Chest radiographs and a CT scan of the cervical region, thorax, abdomen, and pelvis should be performed. Increasingly, disease is being upstaged by PET scan, although its role in staging, restaging, and follow-up of the various lymphomas (especially extranodal marginal zone lymphoma [EMZL] and MALT lymphoma) is still being defined.

Lymphoma treatment has undergone a revolution with the recognition of the role of infectious agents, autoimmune processes, antigenic stimulation, and molecular genetic aberrations in the pathogenesis of lymphoma. Antibiotic treatment of *Helicobacter pylori* in lymphomas associated with gastric MALT has resulted in high resolution rates. Orbital lymphoma has been shown to be associated with *Chlamydia psittaci* in Italy and some other geographic locations, although this has not been replicated in large French and North American studies. This raises the possibility of resolution of the OALD with eradication of the inciting infection/antigen. Oral treatment with doxycycline has had success in Italy but generally not elsewhere. This represents a simple treatment with low morbidity and low cost that might be used initially in geographic locations with a known *Chlamydia* association. Further studies to identify causative agents including *Chlamydia*, Epstein Barr, and hepatitis C are being conducted.

Radiotherapy is regarded as the first-line treatment for localized disease. A dose of 32 cGy has been shown to be over 98% effective in eliminating local disease. There is a very low incidence of local recurrence, but a recognized 10% to 25% rate of systemic involvement in patients with primary OALD over 10-year follow-up. Radiotherapy is also associated with known ocular and adnexal side effects.

Various chemotherapy regimens have also been used, without radiotherapy, and are associated with response rates of 66% to 100%, but have a local recurrence rate of up to 30%.

Another major advance has been the development of monoclonal antibodies to lymphocytes.

Immunotherapy with the antiCD-20 antibody rituximab is being increasingly used in CD-20+ve lymphomas and has been shown to be effective in OALD, usually in combination with conventional chemotherapy. Radioimmunotherapy for OALD is currently being studied prospectively. Response to treatment can be quantitatively assessed by DWI MRI. DWI measures tissue water motion and this can be quantified into an apparent diffusion coefficient (ADC). Increasing ADC suggests a favorable treatment response, whereas a decreasing ADC suggests a negative treatment response.[5]

Long-term follow-up of patients with OALD shows a worse prognosis for patients with lacrimal gland involvement, bilateral disease, or systemic disease at diagnosis. Tumor-related deaths range from 13% for marginal zone lymphoma up to 50% for those with aggressive histologies, including DLBCL, MCL, and T-cell lesions.

Summary

Always consider lymphoma in the differential diagnosis of orbital disease. Have a low threshold for obtaining imaging and biopsy specimens when lymphoma is suspected. Once a diagnosis has been made, consult with an oncologist/hematologist for appropriate staging of the disease and for planning of treatment.

References

1. Coupland SE, White VA, Rootman J, Damato B, Finger PT. A TNM-based clinical staging system of Ocular Adnexal Lymphoma. *Arch Pathol Lab Med.* 2009;133:1262-1267.
2. Ferry JA, Fung CY, Zukerberg L, et al. Lymphoma of the ocular adnexa: a study of 353 cases. *Am J Surg Pathol.* 2007;31:170-184.
3. Jenkins C, Rose GE, Bunce C, et al. Clinical features associated with survival of patients with lymphoma of the ocular adnexa. *Eye.* 2003;17:809-820.
4. Nakayama R, Matsumoto Y, Horiike S, et al. Close pathogenetic relationship between ocular immunoglobulin G4-related disease (IgG4-RD) and ocular adnexal mucosa-associated lymphoid tissue (MALT) lymphoma. *Leuk Lymphoma.* 2014;55(5):1198-1202.
5. Prat MC, Surapaneni K, Chalian H, DeLaPaz RL, Kazim M. Ocular adnexal lymphoma: monitoring response to therapy with diffusion-weighted imaging. *Ophthal Plast Reconstr Surg.* 2013;29:424-427.

SECTION IV

TRAUMA

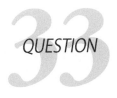
How Do You Treat Children With Orbital Fractures?

Jennifer A. Sivak-Callcott, MD and
John Nguyen, MD

What are the common causes of orbital fracture in children? How and why do orbital fractures differ in children compared to adults? What history is important to illicit and why? What examination should be performed and what findings suggest the need for surgical intervention? How urgently should surgery be undertaken in pediatric orbital fractures and what are the risks?

Orbital fractures in children are rare.[1-3] The most common causes include falls, motor vehicle accidents, assault, and sport-related injury.[2,3] Sport injuries increase in frequency with age, with baseball being the most common cause of orbital fracture.[2,4]

Children have larger craniofacial ratios, with proportionately smaller, flatter midfaces that include a more generous fat pad. Their bones are more elastic, with thicker sinus walls, and less pneumatized frontal sinuses.[1-3] Therefore, orbital roof fractures are most common in children aged younger than 7 years. It is crucial to rule out neurologic injury in these cases because associated intracranial trauma is often present.[3] If there is any evidence of penetrating injury, even subtle eyelid laceration, orbital and intracranial foreign body must by ruled out with imaging, as death from intracranial abscess can occur.

After age 7, floor fractures become increasingly common.[1] These differ from adults in that they are often small, linear, and more likely to entrap orbital tissue. Although the floor is the most common location, medial wall trapdoor fractures have been reported.[5] Unlike adult fractures, these often present with minimal periorbital swelling or ecchymosis, hence the name *white-eyed fracture* (Figure 33-1A).[1]

The mechanism and time of injury, nausea, vomiting, pain, loss of consciousness, change in vision, diplopia, and facial numbness must be recorded. Nausea/vomiting carry a positive predictive value of 75% for trapdoor fracture and 83% for inferior rectus muscle entrapment.[1] Entrapped extraocular muscle can trigger the oculocardiac reflex: the triad of bradycardia, nausea/vomiting,

Kersten RC, McCulley TJ, eds. *Curbside Consultation in Oculoplastics:*
49 Clinical Questions, Second Edition (pp 169-172).
© 2016 Taylor & Francis Group.

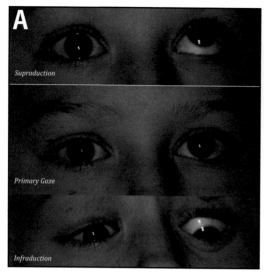

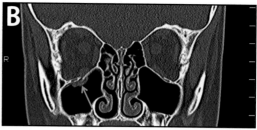

Figure 33-1. (A) Pediatric white-eyed orbital floor fracture demonstrating decreased ability to look up. (B) Coronal CT scan demonstrating small fracture with entrapment (arrow).

and syncope. These can also occur in intracranial injury, and because small orbital fractures with entrapment may not be seen on computed tomography (CT) scan, accurate diagnosis can be delayed or missed (Figure 33-1B).[1]

A full eye exam must be completed. Globe injury, although rare, must be ruled out. Extraocular motility must be carefully documented with special attention to up and lateral movement. Between 44% and 100% of patients with entrapment will have severe restriction.[1] Muscle innervation injury can also be present and will not improve with surgery. If possible, forced ductions should be documented to indicate restrictive strabismus. Globe position, including enophthalmos, vertical or horizontal displacement, orbital hemorrhage, facial sensation, and external edema, ecchymosis, and laceration should be recorded.

Restrictive strabismus, pain, nausea/vomiting, and oculocardiac reflex are highly suggestive for extraocular muscle entrapment, which requires urgent surgical intervention. Children can have white-eyed fractures in which there is minimal edema, negative CT findings, no enophthalmos, but marked extraocular movement restriction (Figure 33-2A). Careful examination is of paramount importance.

Imaging should be performed when there is a history of trauma with clinical evidence of orbital fracture, especially in cases of possible adjacent fracture or foreign body. Noncontrast CT of the orbits is the gold standard for imaging orbital fractures (Figure 33-2B). Due to the risk for significant radiation exposure, pediatric protocols should be used, and multiple scans should be avoided.[1] Magnetic resonance imaging (MRI) using an orbital coil provides excellent images, but requires sedation for younger patients, is more costly, and is not the current standard.[1] Communication of expected findings (small fracture, possibility of entrapment, foreign body) with the radiologist is very important. Concordance rates between radiologic and intraoperative entrapment are only 50% in children vs 87% in adults.[1] Even if the CT scan appears negative for fracture, surgery should be undertaken if there is clinical evidence of entrapment.

In nonentrapped cases, as in adults, we offer elective repair if enophthalmos greater than 2 mm, and/or fracture greater than 50% of the floor is present. In children with entrapped orbital tissue, we feel strongly that they need to be operated on sooner than adults, within 24 to 48 hours.[1] Although there are no prospective randomized trials to determine optimal timing of repair, available evidence shows outcomes are worse when surgery is delayed in the setting of entrapment. The most common complication of fracture repair is persistent diplopia, which is guaranteed if there

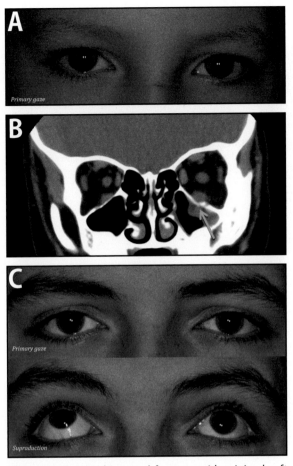

Figure 33-2. (A) White-eyed fracture, with minimal soft tissue signs. (B) Coronal CT scan demonstrating entrapped inferior rectus muscle (arrow). (C) Significant decrease in left eye superior movement.

is a neurogenic component to the strabismus (Figure 33-2C). Infection, hemorrhage, blindness, implant, and anesthesia related risks must be part of the consent process.

Overall, outcomes of orbital fracture are worse in children than adults, which may due to missed or delayed diagnosis. Diplopia can take twice as long to resolve, up to 18 months in some reports.[1] Children aged younger than 9 years have the greatest chance of persistent diplopia, over 50% in some studies, even with complete surgical release of entrapped extraocular muscle.[1] These evidenced-based outcomes must be discussed preoperatively, so that the patient and family have reasonable expectations.

In short, pediatric orbital fractures have a higher likelihood of entrapment, minimal inflammation, and worse outcome, especially if treatment is delayed. Please either treat or refer them to your preferred orbital surgeon urgently.

References

1. Wei LA, Durairaj VD. Pediatric orbital floor fractures. *J AAPOS*. 2011;15(2):173-80. Doi:10.1016/j.jaapos.2011.02.005 PMID:21596296

2. Chapman VM, Fenton LZ, Gao D, Strain JD. Facial fractures in children: unique patterns of injury observed by computed tomography. *J Comput Assist Tomog*. 2009;33(1):70-72. Doi:10.1097/RCT.0b013e318169bfdc PMID:19188788.

3. Joshi S, Kassira W, Thaller SR. Overview of pediatric orbital fractures. *J Craniofac Surg*. 2011;22(4):1330-1332. Doi: 10.1097/SCS.0b013e31821c9365. PMID:21772188.

4. Stotland MA, Do NK. Pediatric orbital fractures. *J Craniofac Surg*. 2011;22(4):1230-1235. Doi:10.1097/SCS.0b013e31821c0f52 PMID:21772209.

5. McCulley TJ, Yip CC, Kersten RC, Kulwin DR. Medial rectus muscle incarceration in pediatric medial orbital wall trapdoor fractures. *Eur J Ophthalmol*. 2004;14(4):330-333. PMID: 15309979.

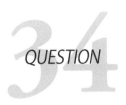

WHAT IMPLANT DO YOU LIKE BEST FOR REPAIRING ORBITAL FRACTURES?

Marc J. Hirschbein, MD, FACS and
Ana Carolina Victoria, MD

What implants are available? Do you use the same implant for children and adults?
The aim of surgical repair of orbital fractures is to prevent enophthalmos and diplopia by restoring normal orbital volume and releasing any entrapped tissue. There are a variety of implant materials that could be used including autogenous, allogenic, and alloplastic. The decision of which material to use to repair a fracture depends on the nature of the fracture, the surgeon's preference, and availability of material at the time of surgery.

The management of orbital fractures has been an active topic of debate for many years, especially as more alloplastic materials are being developed that are better tolerated by the orbital tissues. It is widely accepted that not all orbital fractures require surgical treatment, and for us a 2-week observation period is customary to evaluate the need for surgery. The exception to this rule is the so-called trapdoor fracture in children and young adults, which requires immediate repair. Primary guidelines for orbital fracture repair include enophthalmos of 2 mm or greater, nonresolving diplopia (with tissue entrapment), or large fracture size on imaging (>50% of the floor). Additional indications include hypoglobus or a palpable step-off fracture. Small fractures of the medial orbital wall or floor are usually left untreated because it is thought that the risk for subsequent enophthalmos is low.

Surgical Management of Orbital Fractures

Once the decision to repair has been made, there are different approaches to the orbit: subciliary, mid-lower lid, infraorbital, transconjunctival, and more recently endoscopic. The surgical approach varies within subspecialties as well as comfort level of the surgeon. In our institution,

Kersten RC, McCulley TJ, eds. *Curbside Consultation in Oculoplastics:*
49 Clinical Questions, Second Edition (pp 173-176).
© 2016 Taylor & Francis Group.

Table 34-1
Alloplastic Orbital Implants

Nonporous	Absorbable
Silicone	No
Titanium	No
Polytetrafluoroethylene (Teflon)	No
Nylon	No
Hyaluronate/carboxymethylcellulose	Yes
Polylactide copolymer plates (PLLA, GA, PDS)	Yes
Porous	Absorbable
Porous polyethylene	No
Hydroxyapatite	No
Composite	No

PLLA = poly-L-lactic acid; GA = glycolic acid; PDS = polydioxanone sheets.

we favor the transconjunctival approach (rarely combined with a lateral canthotomy/cantholysis if needed for greater exposure). This incision allows for good visualization of the orbit and for extension of the incision if there is a concomitant medial wall fracture that needs to be repaired. It also allows for an excellent aesthetic result with no visible scar, and it minimizes the likelihood of postoperative lower eyelid retraction.

Orbital Implants

There is a wide array of implant options to be used to repair orbital fractures—from autogenous and allogenic tissues to alloplastic materials. The perfect implant would be biocompatible, easily integrated by the surrounding tissues, have the ability to be molded to a desired shape, and be cost-effective. In the early years of orbital fracture repair, autogenous bone such as cranial bone and iliac bone were used, and are still in use today. Advantages of autogenous bone include biocompatability and availability. Proposed disadvantages include donor site morbidity, increased surgical time, and an unpredictable amount of postoperative resorption.

Many different alloplastic materials have been developed through the years, all with their inherent drawbacks (Table 34-1).[1-4] These implants can be divided into nonporous (eg, silicone, polydiaxonone, polytetrafluoroethylene, nylon, titanium) and porous materials (hydroxyapatite, porous polyethylene). Absorbable implants are also available. Advantages of nonporous implants are availability, cost, and depending on the material, radio-opacity (allowing for easier visualization on computed tomography [CT] scan, as seen with titanium). Reported disadvantages of nonporous materials include increased risk for infection, extrusion, migration, and encapsulation. Proposed advantages of porous materials include tissue integration, lower infection rates, and lower rates of

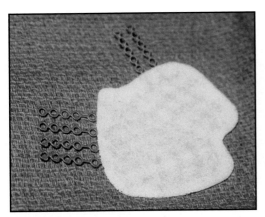

Figure 34-1. Medpor Titan implant.

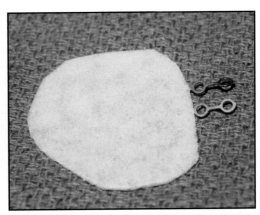

Figure 34-2. Medpor Titan implant after shaping and cutting down to desired size.

extrusion/migration. Disadvantages include cost, availability, and radiolucency (making it hard to evaluate implant position postsurgically). Our implant of choice is a composite implant made of porous polyethylene and titanium called Medpor Titan (Porex Surgical Inc) and Synpor (Synthes) (Figures 34-1 and 34-2). The porous polyethylene face allows for tissue ingrowth and decreases the rate of extrusion. The orbital side of the implant is layered with nonporous polyethylene, decreasing unwanted adhesion to the orbital tissue. The integrated titanium mesh allows for some degree of custom shaping through both bending and cutting. The implant is particularly useful for combined floor and medial wall repairs. The titanium extends beyond the implant, allowing for easier fixation to the maxillary bone outside of the orbit (inferior to the orbital rim). The titanium is also radio-opaque for improved postoperative assessment of plate position. Disadvantages of this implant include cost and availability. If improperly placed (particularly when used for combined floor and medial wall implants), overcorrection and damage to healthy orbital tissue is possible.

For large defects of the orbit and its surrounding structures, such as those seen after resection of malignant tumors and gunshot wounds, there are computer-assisted custom-made three-dimensional implants.[5] They are made of titanium mesh, polyetheretherketones (PEEK), or high-density polyethylene. The implants are made by obtaining three-dimensional imaging of the patient. Once the manufacturer has the images, the implant is made as the mirror image of the unaffected side. The surgeon then receives the implant or a model of the implant, and can shape it preoperatively, therefore decreasing the amount of time spent in the operating room manipulating the implant. These implants still carry the inherent risks for extrusion and infection and can be quite costly.

Considerations in Pediatric Patients

Pediatric patients with orbital floor fractures are a different entity, often requiring urgent surgical repair. Pediatric orbital fractures are usually small, green, stick-type trapdoor fractures that lead to muscle entrapment. Also referred to as the *white-eyed blowout fracture*, the key to management is for the emergency department physician, the radiologist, and the orbital trauma surgeon to maintain a high index of suspicion to avoid delayed diagnosis and potential ischemia to the entrapped muscle. Surgical intervention is more often aimed at releasing the entrapment, as opposed to restoring orbital volume, and rarely to prevent enophthalmos if there is a large fracture. Implants are not always required, as they are reserved in this population for cases with larger fractures or those with greater risk for scarring. Controversies exist regarding choice of implant material. Some authors favor autologous bone grafts. Others advocate absorbable hardware, which include poly-L-lactic acid (PLLA), polyglactin (PGA), glycolic acid (GA), and polydioxanone (PDS) sheets.[4] PLLA has been shown to be better tolerated by the orbital tissues when compared with PGA and PDS. Proposed advantages of these implants include the absence of inhibition to continued bone growth. However, absorbable implants may have a more significant inflammatory reaction. Also, if absorbed before bony regrowth has occurred, the orbital tissues have no support and this may lead to enophthalmos. The composite implants have been used in the pediatric population successfully with no major adverse effects. In our institution, pediatric fractures that require implantation due to increased orbital volume are repaired using composite implants. The implant is secured down to the orbital rim with only one fixation point to avoid interference with future facial bony growth.

Summary

Orbital fractures can have significant disfiguring and dysfunctional effects on the globe if not treated properly or promptly. Although not all fractures need repair, those that do benefit from an implant that will restore volume while allowing for long-term stability and biocompatibility. Obviously, autologous bone is the ideal implant material for reconstruction. However, we feel that the composite implants provide an excellent result with no donor site morbidity and decreased surgical time.

References

1. Aldekhayel S, Aljaaly H, Fouda-Neel O, Shararah AW, Zaid WS, Gilardino M. Evolving trends in the management of orbital floor fractures. *J Craniofac Surg.* 2014;25:258-261.
2. Bratton EM, Durairaj VD. Orbital implants for fracture repair. *Curr Opin Ophthalmol.* 2011;22;400-406.
3. Potter JK, Malmquist M, Ellis E 3rd. Biomaterials for reconstruction of the internal orbit. *Oral Maxillofac Surg Clin North Am.* 2012;24:609-627.
4. Gunarajah DR, Samman N. Biomaterials for repair of orbital floor blowout fractures: a systematic review. *J Oral Maxillofac Surg.* 2013;71:550-570.
5. Frodel J. Computer-designed implants for fronto-orbital defect reconstruction. *Facial Plast Surg.* 2008;24:22-34.

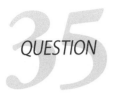

CAN YOU TELL ME ABOUT STEREOTACTIC IMAGE GUIDANCE AND HOW IT IS USED IN ORBITAL SURGERY?

Roger E. Turbin, MD

What is image guidance? Do you find it to be helpful with orbital surgery? If so, for which procedures is it most beneficial?

Image-guided navigational surgery is increasingly applied in the fields of skull base, endoscopic, and otolaryngologic surgery. The most widely available technologies provide real-time precise (1- to 2-mm error), three-dimensional localization of surgical instrument tips relative to preoperatively acquired computed tomography (CT), magnetic resonance imaging (MRI), or fused (CT/MRI) images. The widespread application of navigational surgery and the ability to provide real-time X, Y, and Z plane localization is attractive to the orbital surgeon, yet has current limitations in both technical and conceptual applicability. I will present an overview of basic concepts, and discuss my experience with respect to technical benefits and limits of practical application. So let us begin with some concepts.

Navigational surgery in its purest form could theoretically be experienced in 3 flavors. The first form requires intraoperative dynamic MRI or CT imaging capability, which although expensive, is currently available in some major centers. Theoretically, the surgeon could precisely delineate anatomic regions and pathology in real time in the surgical arena. Over the years, I have participated in combined neurosurgical complex resections of sino-orbito-cranial tumor in which we have used intraoperative open MRI. In general, I have found these procedures to be limited by technologic constraints of relatively low-quality images, and the cumbersome requirement to transfer the open MRI into and out of its shielded housing, and into and out of the surgical field to acquire images, all the while taking great care to maintain the sterility of the operative field and open surgical site. Our particular unit required repositioning of the MRI open magnet into and out of the immediate operative field, which was accomplished by raising the magnet and dropping the magnet around the head, as well as a complete (and expensive) set of MRI-safe surgical instruments and anesthetic cart. We would limit the time-consuming acquisition of images to a few critical intrasurgical assessments to help determine the extent of residual tumor when it

Kersten RC, McCulley TJ, eds. *Curbside Consultation in Oculoplastics:*
49 Clinical Questions, Second Edition (pp 177-181).
© 2016 Taylor & Francis Group.

seemed an appropriate time to scan. Imaging was therefore limited to operative breaks when we could stop the dissection, and imaging was not available easily in real time. In selected cases, it was certainly useful to acquire essentially an interval postoperative scan at a variety of time points and take another shot at removing occult residual tumor without a return to the operating room after wound closure. However, I must admit I agree with one of the neurosurgical residents who whispered, "Oh no, not another one. I hate these cases." One would expect later generations of intraoperative scanners to overcome some of these issues, although likely at significant expense.

The latter two navigational flavors are based on the real-time localization of the tip of a surgical instrument in space, which is imaged as an axial, coronal, and sagittal reconstruction. If intraoperative imaging was available, the rendering could be linked to continually updated intraoperative images. In practice, the images are rendered relative to the baseline preoperatively acquired CT, MRI, or fused images. If dynamic imaging were available, source images would be theoretically updated as the case proceeds. Currently, localization is linked to the presurgical acquired images, and there is no correctional volume rendering as the case progresses and, for instance, a large tumor is resected. Again, the paradigm that employs intraoperative reimaging is currently quite limited, and I will therefore limit further discussion to image-guided techniques based on preoperative baseline images, currently the most widely available technique that today's orbital surgeons most likely employ.

CT and/or MRI images are acquired prior to the scheduled case through protocol specific studies via standard CT or MRI scanners. The images are transferred to a portable computer workstation, which is present in the operative suite. Each of the commercially available surgical systems then use one of a variety of approaches to register and correlate the three-dimensional location of the operative site to the three-dimensional volume rendering of the scan, translated into axial, coronal, and sagittal images in the X, Y, and Z three-dimensional planes. In general, a set of cameras receive an infrared signal that has been registered in space relative to the patient's head. The signal may originate from a set of cameras that act as the transmitter and receiver of signal passively reflected from or actively generated by the surgical instrument of choice. Critical to the system is the ability to register and maintain a rigid and unchanging theoretical three-dimensional volume fixed in space relative to the transmitters and receivers. Also, instruments must be capable of emitting signal or acting as infrared reflectors. These instruments are integrated to the specific system, or options exist to attach infrared reflectors that can be fixed to the distal end of the handle. After the registration is complete, as long as the relationships remain fixed, the system generates real-time axial, coronal, and sagittal maps of the location of the tip of the instrument that is registered to the system (Figure 35-1).

It is in this arena that technologic advances over the last decade have increased the ease of use and precision of these systems. Original systems required bulky head frames fixed relative to the Mayfield or similar head holder that is rigidly pinned to the head/skull. Other systems employ techniques to register three-dimensional space to skin fiducials preplaced in the original scans. Newer systems have refined the registration process by allowing for registration of the surface of head and face in space (Figures 35-2 and 35-3). Each of these systems has its limitations. The registration arm either has to be fixed to the head, or the head has to be rigidly stabilized in space relative to a sensor system arm or frame. In general, the orbital surgeon may not typically employ or be familiar with rigid head pin fixation produced by the head fixation system. In addition, many of the systems that eliminate the need for skull fixation by coupling a sensor to the head are very convenient for an endoscopic surgeon operating in the nonsterile field of the nostril, but simply get in the way of the orbital surgeon. The equipment is expensive and the use of the system requires an additional scan, as well as increased operative time.

In practical terms, I use the navigational systems in selected scenarios, and each has most frequently been employed in conjunction with other surgical services in the most complex cases. In general, these are as follows:

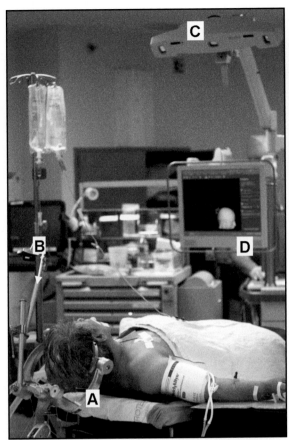

Figure 35-1. The major components of one commercially available navigational system are shown. The patient's head is placed in a rigid fixation system (A) that is coupled to the registration arm (B). The infrared camera (C) reads the location of the registration arm (B), which is fixed in space relative to the head. The location of the head is mapped to the relative location of the registration system, which produces real-time localization of the tip of the instrument in the operative field on the monitor (D).

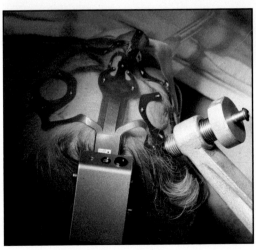

Figure 35-2. A patient surface registration mask is applied, and later removed after successful registration to allow the surgery. The system learns where the surface of the face is rendered in space relative to the registration arm.

- Cases of extensive meningioma involving the skull base and orbital tissue in which surgical landmarks are engulfed by tumor
- Operating in and around the superior/inferior orbital or pterygopalatine fissures (Figure 35-4)

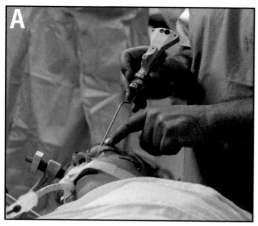 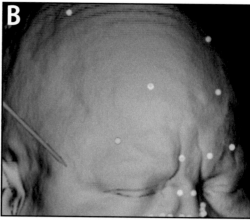

Figure 35-3. (A) The registration pointer is applied to predetermined anatomic landmarks, and volume rendering in space refined using the surgical mask, and the skin surface. (B) These points are translated into the three-dimensional imaging coordinates (MRI, CT, or fused).

Figure 35-4. In this example, an intraoperative surgical pointer (not shown) is applied in the operative field to the medial extent of the dissection of a high-grade meningioma approaching the superior orbital fissure and other elegant structures. The turquoise pointer nicely defines the X, Y, and Z, locations in three-dimensional space rendered by coronal, sagittal, and axial MRIs.

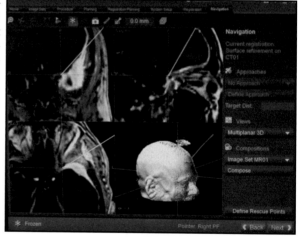

- Near the emergence of the optic nerve from the optic canal in which partial resections are frequently necessary but fragile cranial nerves lie encased within tumor
- Deep orbital bone decompressions in thyroid orbitopathy with optic neuropathy when maximal removal of bone is necessary
- Tumors (frequently cavernous hemangioma) at the orbital apex frequently using a combined intraorbital and endoscopic approach
- Complex sino-orbital lesions in which surgical landmarks have been destroyed by disease process or previous surgery such as allergic fungal aspergillosis.

In soft tissue surgery within the orbit, movement of the orbital contents may limit the utility of real-time localization of the instrument in space. In other words, if the soft tissue moves, the localization will be significantly in error and the navigational rendering does little more than produce a gross anterior posterior estimation. Therefore, I find the navigation most useful when I am working in deep orbital space with relatively fixed lesions, or lesions that are attached/infiltrating bone.

Suggested Readings

Dubin MR, Tabaee A, Scruggs JT, Kazim M, Close LG. Image-guided endoscopic orbital decompression for Graves' orbitopathy. *Ann Otol Rhinol Laryngol*. 2008;117(3):177-185.

Hejazi N. Frameless image-guided neuronavigation in orbital surgery: practical applications. *Neurosurg Rev*. 2006;23;29(2):118-122.

Hodaj I, Kutlay M, Gonul E, et al. The use of neuronavigation and intraoperative imaging systems in the surgical treatment of orbital tumors. *Turk Neurosurg*. 2014;24(4):549-557.

Servat JJ, Elia MD, Gong D, Manes RP, Black EH, Levin F. Electromagnetic image-guided orbital decompression: technique, principles, and preliminary experience with 6 consecutive cases. *Orbit*. 2014;33(6):433-436.

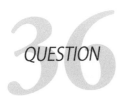

WHAT IS TRAUMATIC OPTIC NEUROPATHY?

Stuart R. Seiff, MD, FACS

What is the mechanism of injury of indirect traumatic optic neuropathy? How should I evaluate a patient with presumed traumatic optic neuropathy? What happens to patients who are not treated? What kind of treatment can we offer patients? What is the role of medical treatment? What is the role for surgical decompression of the optic canal? What treatment should I offer patients with traumatic optic neuropathy?

Injuries to the optic nerve may occur in a direct or indirect fashion. Direct injuries are usually not subtle, typically arising as a result of penetration of the orbit by foreign bodies, missiles, penetrating stab wounds, bone fragments, or fractures extending through the optic canal. Vision loss is usually severe and, in most cases, no effective therapy is available for this type of injury.

Indirect traumatic optic neuropathy typically occurs in the setting of blunt frontal trauma in which a moving head suddenly decelerates with impact in the region of the brow or forehead. Vision loss is noted in the presence of an otherwise normal eye. The visual acuity may be slightly or severely decreased, frequently to no light perception levels. An afferent pupil defect may be the only objective finding because the optic nerve appearance is typically normal upon early examination. With time, optic atrophy will develop.

Indirect traumatic optic neuropathy most frequently occurs in motor vehicle and bicycle accidents, assaults, and falls, with the final common pathway being blunt frontal trauma. The exact mechanism of optic nerve injury is poorly studied. Holographic interferometry has suggested that the energy from the blow is transmitted to the region of the optic canal. This is consistent with the finding that the intracanalicular portion of the optic nerve is commonly the site of injury. However, other sections of the optic nerve are occasionally involved and other factors may be at play.

Evaluation should begin with assessment of visual acuity. When possible, the vision should be monitored closely, as postinjury deterioration has been reported. Unfortunately, this may be

Kersten RC, McCulley TJ, eds. *Curbside Consultation in Oculoplastics:*
49 Clinical Questions, Second Edition (pp 183-185).
© 2016 Taylor & Francis Group.

Figure 36-1. Large displaced bony fragment of the orbit apex seen in a patient with a traumatic optic neuropathy.

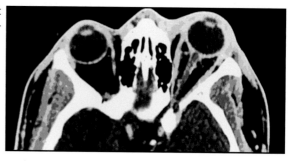

difficult given the severity of the associated injuries. The patient should be tested for an afferent pupillary defect, the most indicative finding of optic nerve injury. Associated orbital and cranial nerve trauma should also be evaluated. Multiple cranial neuropathies may indicate severe skull base pathology and possible involvement of the carotid artery. Patterns of visual field loss vary widely, but typically include central depression, which accounts for the decreased acuity. Of course, ocular injury should be assessed in all trauma patients.

I recommend that all patients suspected of having a traumatic optic neuropathy undergo urgent fine cut computed tomography (CT) scanning to evaluate both the brain and the orbit. Fine cut direct coronal or reconstructed images through the optic canal are needed to identify fractures in this area. Fractures of the optic canal and adjacent structures are frequently present but are not necessary to make the diagnosis (Figure 36-1).

Several studies have looked at visual acuity in patients who do not undergo treatment. It appears that 20% to 50% of cases will have some degree of spontaneous recovery of visual acuity.[1,2] More recent experiences also suggest that improvement is often early (within 5 to 7 days). This would account for the underestimation of spontaneous improvement rates in reports comprised of late referral patients. Despite the potential for spontaneous improvement, in my experience, significant recovery to near-normal vision is rare.

Treatment has focused on managing theoretically reversible components of the injury (eg, edema and inflammation), both medically with corticosteroids, as well as surgically with optic canal decompression. Corticosteroid use has been common since the early 1980s. Several anecdotal studies showed improvement in visual acuity with corticosteroids.[1,3] The initial theory was that these drugs reduced edema of the nerve within the optic canal, reducing compression. However, the current rationale for corticosteroid use is that, among other things, they may inhibit oxygen-free radical-induced lipid peroxidation and decrease the degree of vasospasm.

These theories arise from work on spinal cord injuries. The National Acute Spinal Cord Injury Study (NASCIS) 2 and 3 trials suggested that methylprednisolone given as a bolus of 30 mg/kg, intravenously, followed by 5.4 mg/kg per hour for 48 hours, had improved neurologic function after spinal cord injury.[4] Although it is recognized that spinal cord and optic nerve injuries have several important differences, this regimen was recommended for the management of indirect traumatic optic neuropathy. No study has been completed with this as the primary treatment approach. Moreover, steroid efficacy has more recently been called into question as patients in the NASCIS studies were found to have only limited neurologic recovery over time, and there were indications of increased life-threatening infections after steroid use. Additionally, the CRASH study further elucidated complications of steroid use in head injuries.[5] Available data have shown that the risk-to-benefit ratio is particularly unfavorable if steroids are not administered within 8 hours of injury. Thus, the initial enthusiasm for steroid use in traumatic optic neuropathy has been somewhat suppressed.

Surgical decompression of the optic canal is also advocated by some. The goal of surgical decompression of the optic nerve within the optic canal has been the release of compression by removing bone around an edematous nerve, possibly improving vascular perfusion. Again, there are anecdotal reports of some success with this approach, but the overall positive effect seems quite low.[6] Also, in the best controlled study assessing optic nerve decompression (IONTS), no benefit was seen.[2] One exception where I might recommend surgical decompression is in a patient with a fracture involving and compromising the optic canal.

Unfortunately, there remain no randomized controlled trials for traumatic optic neuropathy comparing the outcomes between observation, high-dose corticosteroids, and surgical decompression of the optic canal. One study, the IONTS, was a comparative nonrandomized interventional study with concurrent treatment groups that compared the visual outcome in patients with indirect traumatic optic neuropathy treated with corticosteroids, optic canal decompression, or observation alone.[2] After adjustment for baseline vision, there were no significant differences between any of the treatment groups. In fact, although not statistically significant, untreated patients had greater rates of improvement than those treated with steroids or surgery. Although this study was not sufficiently powered to exclude all treatment benefit, I believe that it does rule out major effects. Another important finding of this study was the confirmation that there is spontaneous early improvement, without treatment, in many patients felt to have a traumatic optic neuropathy. This is important to remember when evaluating rates of improvement in prior studies.

Summary

Based on the existing literature, neither corticosteroids nor optic canal surgery should be considered the standard of care for patients with traumatic optic neuropathy. It is reasonable for clinicians to use their judgment to decide how to treat an individual patient. If seen acutely (within 8 hours of injury), I occasionally recommend the use of steroids and follow the guidelines outlined by the NASCIS studies. Rarely do I recommend surgical decompression of the optic canal.

References

1. Seiff SR. High dose corticosteroids for treatment of vision loss due to indirect injury to the optic nerve. *Ophthalmic Surg.* 1990;21:389-395.
2. Levin LA, Beck RW, Joseph MP, Seiff S, Kraker R. The treatment of traumatic optic neuropathy: the International Optic Nerve Trauma Study. *Ophthalmology.* 1999;106:1268-1277.
3. Anderson RL, Panje WR, Gross CE. Optic nerve blindness following blunt forehead trauma. *Ophthalmology.* 1982;80:445-455.
4. Bracken MB, Shepard MJ, Holford TR, et al. Methylprednisolone or tirilazad mesylate administration after acute spinal cord injury: 1-year follow up. Results of the third National Acute Spinal Cord Injury randomized controlled trial. *J Neurosurg.* 1998;89:699-706.
5. Edwards P, Arango M, Balica L, et al. Final results of MRC CRASH, a randomised placebo-controlled trial of intravenous corticosteroid in adults with head injury-outcomes at 6 months. *Lancet.* 2005;365(9475):1957-1959.
6. Levin LA, Joseph MP, Rizzo JF III, Lessel S. Optic canal decompression in indirect optic nerve trauma. *Ophthalmology.* 1994;101:566-569.

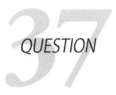

WHAT SHOULD I DO FOR
AN ORBITAL HEMORRHAGE?

Michael Kazim, MD and
Payal Patel, MD

What is the risk for an orbital hemorrhage with blepharoplasty? Should I perform a canthotomy and cantholysis? If so, when? Is the management similar for hemorrhages due to different causes? At what point should a patient be taken to the operating room?

Orbital hemorrhages can occur in a variety of clinical settings. Most commonly, they result from blunt or penetrating trauma or after surgery—both deep orbital and superficial cosmetic eyelid surgery. Self-limited, functionally insignificant orbital hemorrhages are commonly encountered during surgery. Vision threatening hemorrhage, however, is rare. The incidence of orbital hemorrhage following blepharoplasty has been reported as 1 in 2000 and the incidence of significant visual loss following blepharoplasty has been reported to be 1 in 10,000. (Figure 37-1).[1,2] Most hemorrhages in this setting typically occur within 24 hours of surgery but can occur as late as 1 week following surgery.

The clinical signs of orbital hemorrhage include pain, proptosis, limited ocular motility, resistance to retropulsion, increased intraocular pressure, and, if severe, optic neuropathy heralded by decreased visual acuity, afferent pupil defect, and compromise of retinal perfusion. The cause of vision loss is usually an increase in orbital pressure above mean arterial pressure in the arteries supplying the optic nerve or retina; rarely, marked axial prolapse of the globe may result in stretch optic neuropathy. Although the time interval for vision preservation may vary and is dependent on a number of variables—including the age and general health of the patient—the best prospects for recovery of vision occur within 90 minutes of the hemorrhage.[3]

The initial intervention should include both lateral canthotomy and cantholysis of the lower and upper eyelids. Releasing the eyelids temporally from their attachment to the orbital periosteum produces a rapid reduction in the orbital pressure.[4,5] For a hemorrhage following surgery, the wounds should be opened to drain trapped blood. If effective, these maneuvers should result in a

Kersten RC, McCulley TJ, eds. *Curbside Consultation in Oculoplastics:*
49 Clinical Questions, Second Edition (pp 187-190).
© 2016 Taylor & Francis Group.

Figure 37-1. Orbital hemorrhage following 4-eyelid blepharoplasty. Hemorrhaging was present bilaterally, but to a greater degree on the left, resulting in a loss of vision to no light perception.

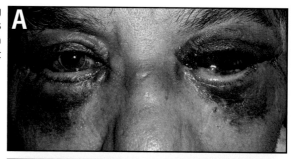

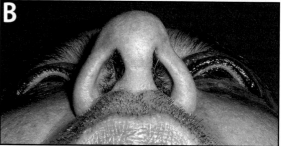

decrease in resistance to retropulsion and improvement in ocular perfusion. Intraocular pressure reflects orbital pressure in this setting and should be monitored with a goal of reducing the pressure to less than 40 mm Hg.

We like to admit patients for observation. They are placed on bed rest with the head elevated and ice compresses applied. Additional medical maneuvers include the administration of diuretics including mannitol and Osmoglyn (glycerin). Diamox (acetazolamide), if tolerated, can be used to a maximum dose of 2 g. Corticosteroids further reduce orbital edema and may be of benefit if the vision fails to improve. The dose of corticosteroids is controversial; however, my preference is 500 to 1000 mg of methylprednisolone daily for 24 to 48 hours. If the hemorrhage occurred as a consequence of minor trauma (Figure 37-2) that normally would not be expected to cause significant hemorrhaging, then the patient's coagulation state should be evaluated. This should include at minimum PT, PTT, and platelet count. Consider consulting a hematologist to assess for genetic or other defects in coagulation. Patients should also be thoroughly questioned as to their use of aspirin or aspirin-containing products, or other nonprescribed medicinal or homeopathic agents that may prolong bleeding times. Coagulation parameters should be normalized by supplementation with platelets or frozen plasma as appropriate.

The recovery of vision should be rapid if the intervention is timely and effective. Complete improvement is anticipated over a period of 1 to 2 weeks. Ocular motility also improves rapidly after decompression, but may take up to several months to recover completely. The canthotomy should be left open for about 1 week to permit resolution of the orbital edema, after which the canthal angle can be reconstructed.

If the canthotomy, cantholysis, and medical measures are ineffective at relieving orbital pressure and optic nerve dysfunction, the patient should be taken to the operating room as expeditiously as possible for orbital exploration, drainage of persistent hemorrhage, and coagulation of arterial bleeding (under general anesthesia). The surgical approach can be made through the original skin and conjunctival wounds if the patient is postsurgery, or through standard orbital approaches if the hemorrhage is due to trauma. In cases where the site of the hemorrhage is not clear, a decompression may be beneficial. In the case of orbital hemorrhage during endonasal sinus surgery, endonasal decompression of the orbit with release of the periorbita can provide immediate relief.

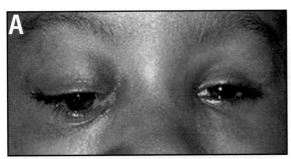

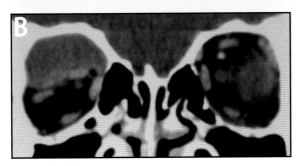

Figure 37-2. Orbital hemorrhage following minor trauma. This child suffered from a subgaleal bleed when his hair was pulled, which tracked down into the right orbit. When significant hemorrhaging is seen following minor trauma, evaluation for a clotting abnormality should be undertaken.

If the hemorrhage is intraconal, axial proptosis and optic nerve stretch may not be improved by canthotomy/cantholysis. If suspected, intraconal blood should be decompressed by direct exploration. If time permits, a CT scan (without contrast) will localize pockets of hemorrhage and assist in constructing a surgical approach.

Spontaneous hemorrhages rarely result from sudden elevation of cranial venous pressure. This includes minor disturbances such as vigorous sneezing, vomiting, or it can be associated with maternal labor or barotraumas. Hemotologic disorders, excessive alcohol intake, and prior orbital surgery are predisposing factors to spontaneous subperiosteal hemorrhage. These typically occur in the superior subperiosteal space at the site of fine perforating vessels. This location is unfortunately commonly associated with optic nerve compression and often requires surgical drainage.[6]

Finally, orbital lesions can bleed spontaneously. These include arteriovenous malformations, lymphangiomas, varices, and more rarely rapidly growing malignant tumors. Among these lesions, lymphangiomas are most likely to produce spontaneous hemorrhage and they are typically managed by the medical means mentioned above. If these are inadequate, then the location of the hemorrhage, so-called chocolate cyst, can be identified by CT or MRI and can be drained to relieve optic nerve compression or exposure-related corneal ulceration. Drainage can be accomplished by either open surgical exploration or by percutaneous CT-guided needle aspiration. Varices and arterial venous malformations require extensive preoperative planning and thrombosis of the lesions prior to surgical intervention.

Summary

Orbital hemorrhages are encountered in a number of clinical settings. Many are self-limiting and require no intervention. When visual loss is encountered, initial management consists of a canthotomy and cantholysis. Unfortunately, in the setting of continued bleeding, the benefits of this maneuver are only temporary. Definitive surgical treatment may involve exploration with coagulation/ligation of the offending blood vessels, removal/drainage of a hematoma, and as a last resort, decompression of the orbit. Do not forget that those occurring with minor trauma warrant clinical assessment for coagulation abnormalities.

References

1. Waller RR. Is blindness a realistic complication of blepharoplasty procedures? *Ophthalmology.* 1978;85:730-735.
2. Hass AN, Penne RB, Stefanyszyn MA, Flanagan JC. Incidence of postblepharoplasty orbital hemorrhage and associated visual loss. *Ophthal Plast Reconstr Surg.* 2004;20:426-432.
3. Nicholson DH. Induced ocular hypertension during photocoagulation of afferent artery in angiomatosis retiane. *Retina.* 1983;3:59.
4. Zoumalan CI, Bullock JD, Warwar RE, Fuller B, McCulley TJ. Evaluation of intraocular and orbital pressure in the management of orbital hemorrhage. *Arch Ophthalmol.* 2008;126(9):1257-1260.
5. Wilcsek JA, Kazim M, Francis INC, et al. Acute orbital hemorrhage. In: Holck DE, Ng JD, eds. *Evaluation and Treatment of Orbital Fractures.* Philadelphia, PA: Elsevier Saunders; 2006:381-389.
6. Elia MD, Shield D, Kazim M, et al. Spontaneous subperiosteal orbital hemorrhage. *Orbit.* 2013;32(5):333-335.

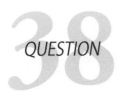
How Should Canalicular Lacerations Be Managed?

Louise A. Mawn, MD, FACS

Should I repair a superior canalicular laceration? How quickly does a canalicular laceration need to be repaired and what technique do you recommend?

Canalicular lacerations are treated surgically. Suspicion that the canaliculus is lacerated should be high in any lid trauma. Either blunt or penetrating injury to the periocular area can disrupt the lacrimal system. To determine if the canaliculus is involved, close examination must be performed, particularly if there are signs of injury at the medial lid. A common dictum is that in any laceration medial to the pupil, the canaliculus is involved until proven otherwise. A careful history detailing the nature of the trauma, the object striking the lid and a complete eye exam to rule out any trauma to the globe should be documented. The tetanus status needs to be confirmed and updated if necessary. If the laceration resulted from an animal bite, the rabies risk must also be assessed and rabies prophylaxis given if the needed.

In most adults and many children, determination of whether the injury involves the canaliculus can be made either in the emergency department or clinic setting by carefully inspecting the lid margin. If uncertainty exists, further confirmation can be obtained by probing and irrigating the lacrimal system; however, if by visible examination the lacrimal system is lacerated, probing at the bedside provides little if any benefit (Figure 38-1) as repair will need to be performed; minimizing any unnecessary manipulation of the lid is beneficial. In small children when the eyelid laceration will need to be repaired under general anesthesia further defining the extent of the injury can be performed in the operating room. Surgical repair can be performed under local anesthesia augmented by intravenous sedation or general anesthesia directed by the extent of the trauma and the comfort and cooperation of the patient.

Reestablishing the anatomy of the medial lid and lacrimal system improves both the aesthetic and functional outcome of the eyelid. Understanding the complex anatomy of the medial lid is

Kersten RC, McCulley TJ, eds. *Curbside Consultation in Oculoplastics:
49 Clinical Questions, Second Edition* (pp 191-195).
© 2016 Taylor & Francis Group.

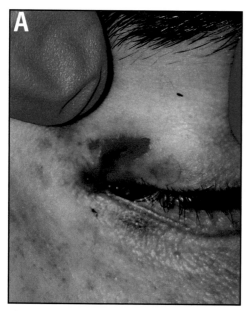 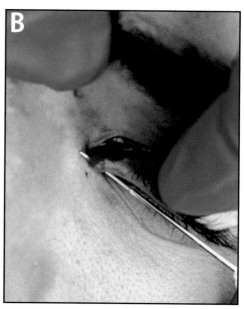

Figure 38-1. (A) A 17-year-old male sustained a laceration of the left upper eyelid while playing basketball. The lacrimal portion of the eyelid is clearly involved. (B) Probing the lacerated canaliculus does not add to the clinical decision making.

paramount in reestablishing function of the lacrimal drainage system. The majority of the lid, the palpebral segment, has lashes and is supported by the tarsal plates. The medial most portion of the lid, the lacrimal segment is free of lashes and is more vulnerable to trauma. The lacrimal system begins at the transition of the palpebral and lacrimal lid. The junction of the squared off palpebral segment of the lid with the more rounded lacrimal portion of the lid, is marked by the slight mound of the upper and lower lid puncta. The puncta are normally slightly turned in against the globe. The 2-mm, vertically oriented puncta makes a slightly less than 90-degree medial turn to the horizontally oriented canaliculus. In the medial 8 mm of the lid, the canaliculus runs immediately beneath the skin and a small strip of orbicularis. The upper and lower canaliculus continue in a posterior medial direction to join behind the anterior limb of the medial canthal tendon and then into the lacrimal sac. Some lacerations will simply involve a laceration to the canaliculus; however, when the lid is avulsed from its medial insertion both the medial canthal tendon and the canaliculus need to be repaired along with the lid margin.

I'm often asked whether superior canalicular lacerations really need to be repaired. In my opinion, all superior canaliculus should be repaired. Repair reestablishes the functional component of the tear drainage system, but equally important, is that when the anatomy is properly restored, the aesthetic appearance of the lid is restored. If the surgical repair does not take into account alignment of the correct layers of the lid, unsightly scarring as well as tearing often results (Figure 38-2). The contribution of both the superior and inferior canaliculus have been demonstrated with tear flow studies.[1-4] Some individuals may drain tears satisfactorily through either the upper or lower canaliculus when the other is blocked, while others may not.[1,2] Symptomatic tearing results from a mismatch of tear production to tear draining capacity. Thus, traumatic loss of a single canaliculus does not necessarily lead to symptoms of tearing.[5,6] However, when faced with an isolated canalicular laceration (upper or lower) there is no way of telling if the patient will be symptom free with one functioning canaliculus.[1] There may be symptoms in up to 50%.[1,2] Medicolegal issues could also potentially arise in patients who experience symptomatic tearing following an eyelid

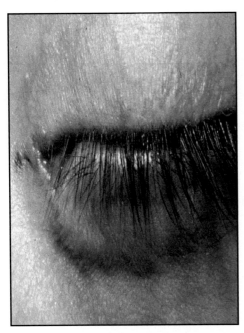

Figure 38-2. A young female injured during a domestic violence assault. The injury to the lacrimal system was unrecognized by the emergency health care provider who repaired the laceration which resulted in both unsightly scarring and loss of normal tear outflow.

injury, who find that no attempt was made to repair their isolated canaliculus laceration.[6] The only way to avoid symptomatic patients is to repair all canalicular lacerations.[1]

In all eyelid lacerations immediate emergency examination should be performed with attention to the globe as well as the ocular adnexa. Immediate gentle cleaning of the wound should be accomplished in the emergency department setting. Cleaning the wound is of paramount importance to decreasing the risk for infection. Povidine-iodine solution 1% to 5% can be instilled over the injured tissue and let to remain in contact with the tissue for 5 minutes. If the wound is contaminated either with soil, debris, or animal saliva, additional gentle irrigation with saline or an antibiotic saline solution should be performed. Any avulsed tissue should be reposited into its normal anatomic location. Antibiotic coverage for the related pathogens should also begin immediately with both topical ophthalmic solution and ointment. If soil contamination is an issue, coverage of *Bacillus cereus* with clindamycin may be needed. There is controversy regarding the use of systemic antibiotics in some injuries including animal bites; however, all canalicular lacerations extend through the dermis and require surgical repair placing these injuries in the high risk for infection category.[7,8] Animal bites typically involve a wide range of bacteria and broad spectrum antibiotics such as amoxicillin/clavulanic acid should begin immediately and continued for 3 to 5 days (Figure 38-3). Also in the setting of a dog bite, evaluation for deeper crushing injury with computed tomography imaging may be needed, especially in a toddler.[9] The earlier an animal bite is cleaned and repaired the better. For the non-animal bite, eyelid lacerations, canalicular repair within 24 to 72 hours can result in excellent functional and aesthetic outcomes (Figure 38-4). There are many techniques for repairing a lacerated canaliculus, but the most important factor is stenting of the lumen of the torn canaliculus. An eloquent, experimental, animal model comparing repair with and without silicone intubation in sheep, showed that silicone intubation was necessary to reestablish patency of the lacrimal system as assessed by probing and histopathologic evaluation.[10] This study also compared tube removal at 4, 8, and 12 weeks and found that 12 weeks was the optimal time for reestablishing patency.[10]

Repair of the canaliculus is best performed by a surgeon, typically an ophthalmologist, familiar with the anatomy of the lacrimal drainage system and the medial eyelid. Local anesthesia with lidocaine and epinephrine can facilitate this repair. To repair the canaliculus, both the proximal

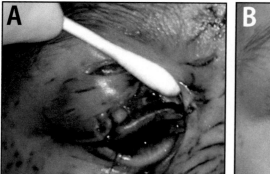
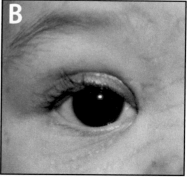

Figure 38-3. (A) A 5-month-old baby injured from an animal attack with involvement of the lacrimal system. (B) A round-eyed pigtail probe facilitated restoration of the lacrimal system.

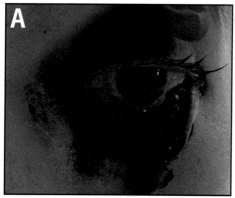
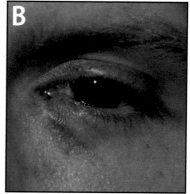

Figure 38-4. (A) A 21-year-old male with complex injury of the ocular adnexa involving the lacrimal system. (B) Repair of lacerations and lacrimal system resulted in a functional tearing system.

and distal end must be identified. Visualization of the delicate white cuff of the lacerated canaliculus requires either surgical loops or microscopic magnification. Illumination from a headlight or microscope also aids this identification. The tissue should be delicately approached with manipulation limited to avoid distorting the anatomy with swelling and bleeding. Surgeons should rely on the lacrimal techniques that they are familiar with when restoring the lacrimal anatomy. Although I personally enjoy the benefits gained from using the round-tipped eyed pigtail probe, this technique has a learning curve and is best used by those surgeons trained in its correct rotational and directional passage through the lacrimal system. The technical steps of canalicular repair with the round-tipped eyed pigtail probe are similar to repair using nasolacrimal stents with a few subtle variations (Figure 38-5).[11] The puncta (if intact) are first dilated with the punctal dilator. The pigtail probe is gently passed through the distal portion of the canalicular system. The eyed tip of the pigtail probe exits the severed portion of the canalicular system. A 6-0 Prolene or nylon suture is then threaded through the eye and rotated back through the distal system. The thread is released from the probe and the probe passed through the opposite side of the lacerated system. When the probe is passed into the medial canthus a slight rotation change in the position of the probe is made as it is passed deep to the medial canthal tendon and then back up again into the opposite canalicular system. The pigtail probe eye is then again threaded with the suture in the proximal portion of the lacerated canalicular system. Once the entire canalicular system is threaded, a small piece, about 24 mm, of silicone stent (Crawford)

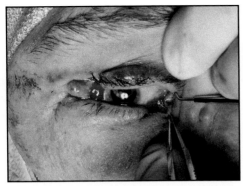

Figure 38-5. Intraoperative photograph of the right eye of a 48-year-old woman who was bitten by a pit bull. The round-eyed pigtail probe is passed through the superior system to facilitate repair of the lacerated inferior canalicular system.

is passed over the suture. The canalicular system is then intubated with the stent by passing it over the suture. The suture is tied, the knot trimmed and the knot is rotated into the intact portion of the canalicular system. The advantage of the stenting accomplished by the pigtail probe technique is that it allows for a casting of the medial lid anatomy.[11] However, the most important factor in canalicular repair is the luminal stenting and this can be accomplished by mono- or bicanalicular stenting. In some instances, mucosal repair with 7-0 polyglactin 910 sutures also augments this closure. If the medial canthal tendon is severed, I use a 4-0 polyglactin 910 suture on a P-2 curved needle to resecure the tendon deep in the medial canthus. I close the lid margin with 7-0 polyglactin 910 sutures. Commonly an extension of the laceration along the nasojugular fold occurs and this component of the laceration can be repaired with simple interrupted closure using 6-0 plain suture. Excellent functional and aesthetic outcomes can be achieved by reestablishing the lacrimal drainage system.

Summary

Lacerations medial to the pupil commonly involve the canaliculus. All canalicular lacerations should be repaired. Optimal repair of a lacerated canaliculus is accomplished by silicone stenting of the lumen for at least 12 weeks.

References

1. Linberg JV, Moore CA. Symptoms of monocanalicular obstruction. *Ophthalmology.* 1988;95:1077-1079.
2. Canavan YM, Archer DB. Long-term review of injuries to the lacrimal drainage apparatus. *Trans Ophthalmol Soc UK.* 1979;99:201-204.
3. Jones LT, Marquis MM, Vincent NJ. Lacrimal functions. *Am J Ophthalmol.* 1972;73:658-659.
4. Lemp MA, Weiler HH. How do tears exit? *Invest Ophthalmol Vis Sci.* 1983;24:616-622.
5. Meyer DR, Antonello A, Linberg JV. Assessment of tear drainage after canalicular obstruction using fluorescein dye disappearance. *Ophthalmology.* 1990;97:1370-1374.
6. Reifler DM. Management of canalicular laceration. *Surv Ophthalmol.* 1991;36(2):113-132.
7. Rui-feng C, Li-song H, Ji-bo Z, Li-qiu W. Emergency treatment on facial laceration of dog bite wounds with immediate primary closure: a prospective randomized trial study. *BMC Emerg Med.* 2013;13(Suppl 1):S2.
8. Esposito S, Picciollo I, Semino M, Principi N. Dog and cat bite-associated infections in children. *Eur J Clin Microbiol Infect Dis.* 2013;32(8):971-976.
9. Wei LA, Chen HH, Hink EM, Durairaj VD. Pediatric facial fractures from dog bites. *Ophthal Plast Reconstr Surg.* 2013;29(3):179-182.
10. Conlon MR, Smith KD, Cadera W, Shum D, Allen LH. An animal model studying reconstruction techniques and histopathological changes in repair of canalicular lacerations. *Can J Ophthalmol.* 1994;30(1):3-8.
11. Jordan DR, Gilberg S, Mawn LA. The round-tipped, eyed pigtail probe for canalicular intubation: a review of 228 patients. *Ophthal Plast Reconstr Surg.* 2008;24(3):176-180.

SECTION V

LACRIMAL

DRAINAGE SYSTEM

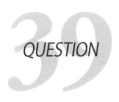

WHAT IS NEW IN THE MANAGEMENT OF ADULT TEARING PATIENTS?

Daniel G. Ezra, MA, MBBS, MMedEd, MD, FRCS, FRCOphth and
Geoffrey E. Rose, BSc, MBBS, MS, DSc, MRCP, FRCS, FRCOphth

Do you have any tips for performing a dacryocystorhinostomy? Is stenting really necessary? Do all patients respond the same to surgery? Do you ever use Jones tubes?

Lacrimal surgery has progressed since appreciation of the dichotomy of symptoms and signs—with volume and flow characteristics having a great relevance in assessing lacrimal problems and gauging the outcome of treatment. Recent emphasis on the importance of complete effacement of the lacrimal sac during dacryocystorhinostomy (DRC), rather than just creating a small opening, has resulted in markedly improved outcomes, with recognition that 100% cure of volume symptoms and signs is achievable. Complete opening of the posterior mucosal flaps is readily achievable only if anterior ethmoidectomy is performed during lacrimal surgery, and recent advances in endonasal techniques have focused on bone removal posteriorly and superiorly—the latter bone to widely expose the common canalicular opening.

Silicone intubation should now be recognized as an epithelial policeman, preventing adhesion of surfaces where there has been mucosal damage, and not as a means of preventing fibrotic closure of an inadequately sized soft tissue anastomosis after DCR. Such intubation should, therefore, be left in place for only the short time required for epithelial healing. New variants of glass canalicular bypass tubes have been hailed as reducing spontaneous tube loss, but these variants generally increase biofilm accumulation, with a secondary inflammatory response, risk for granuloma formation, and tube extrusion.

Kersten RC, McCulley TJ, eds. *Curbside Consultation in Oculoplastics:
49 Clinical Questions, Second Edition* (pp 199-203).
© 2016 Taylor & Francis Group.

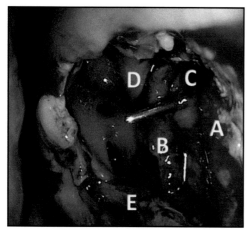

Figure 39-1. Endonasal view of left endoscopic DCR. (A) The reflected anterior lacrimal sac flap. (B) The reflected short posterior sac flap. (C) The opened fundus of sac with 2 to 3 mm clearance of the internal opening. (D) The opened agger nasi air cell, with ethmoidal mucosa in edge-to-edge contact with the posterior mucosa of the lacrimal sac. (E) The trimmed nasal mucosa placed to abut the inferior extent of the opened lacrimal sac mucosa.

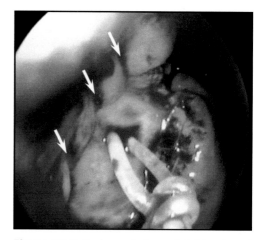

Figure 39-2. Endonasal view of right external DCR: Continuous suturing of the posterior flaps is readily evident, and the arrows indicate the 3 suture sites for the anterior mucosal anastomosis. The sutured flaps ensure complete efface-ment of the lacrimal sac into the nasal mucosa, with no residual sac cavity to form a sump.

Technique

DCR is commonly performed by the oculoplastic surgeon and, although the fundamental principles remain unchanged, many refinements have been made over the years. The key objective of DCR is to maintain an enduring anastomosis between the lacrimal sac and the nose; rather than this being a small opening, it should be recognized that the entire sac needs to be completely effaced into the nasal mucosa (Figures 39-1 and 39-2). This effacement can present technical difficulties that require a detailed anatomical understanding of the lacrimal sac and its adjacent structures if surgery is to be successful.

Variable ethmoidal anatomy, with the anterior air cells often lying alongside the sac fossa, is a common cause for a poor anastomosis and subsequent DCR failure. Such intrusive ethmoidal cells will be found in up to 90% of patients and, without adequate attention to removing these air cells, the posterior reflection of sac mucosa is limited, with a significant risk for retained debris in an unopened sac remnant (sump syndromes; either a high or low sump). Anterior ethmoidectomy should routinely be performed during external DCR to allow unrestricted opening of the poste-rior lacrimal and nasal mucosal flaps. The ethmoidal cells can also be removed during endonasal DCR, or de-roofed and opened, with a short posterior flap fashioned during endonasal DCR to prevent formation of a concave, or birdbox, anastomosis (see Figure 39-1).

Removal of the anterior lacrimal crest during external DCR allows fashioning of a large nasal mucosal flap and wide anterior opening of the sac. Removal of the anterior crest and frontal pro-cess of the maxilla should be emulated with endonasal DCR to allow the anterior sac flap to roll forward and prevent cleft formation around a sac remnant. This often requires drilling or punch-ing out the bone to expose the orbicularis fibers.

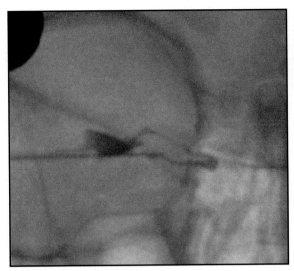

Figure 39-3. Right injection dacryocystogram 3 months after DCR, showing medial common canalicular obstruction at the common internal opening. Note the reflux of contrast through the upper canaliculus and absence of flow into the nose.

Provided the anterior limb of the canthal tendon is divided, external DCR has the advantage of mobilizing the lacrimal sac fundus and thereby allows complete removal of neighboring bone. Although more difficult, removal of the frontal beak overlying the sac can be achieved during powered endonasal DCR—at least to the extent that the common opening is exposed (and ideally to the top of the fundus).

Controlled mucosal healing prevents vigorous fibrosis and is best achieved by ensuring that the soft tissue anastomosis heals by primary, rather than secondary, intention. With external DCR, this is readily accomplished by suturing the flaps (see Figure 39-2), but the secondary intention healing of endonasal DCR can be minimized by good epithelial contact between the lacrimal sac, nasal, and ethmoidal mucosae. The nasal mucosa should be shaped to fit the reflected lacrimal sac flaps, bare areas minimized, and, in some cases, the ethmoidal mucosa can have direct mucosal contact with the posterior sac flap (see Figure 39-1).

Role of Intubation

Silicone intubation, first described by Gibbs,[1] is widely used in DCR, and there has been recent interest in whether it improves outcomes. Although there is a popular and incorrect belief that intubation keeps the soft tissue anastomosis open, the role of intubation is actually to prevent epithelial closure at canalicular level, particularly at the common canalicular opening where adhesions at Rosenmuller's valve can cause postoperative failure (Figure 39-3). Tubes also provide an effective fixation for absorbable nasal packings, and can splint open unsutured flaps or tamponade raw surfaces. These uses are particularly valuable with the secondary intention healing of endonasal surgery.

Although a recent randomized, controlled trial failed to show a difference in outcomes with or without intubation for endonasal DCR,[2] reported success rates for DCR without intubation are as low as 74%. In our opinion, there is currently insufficient evidence to negate the short-term use of intubation.

Symptoms Can Predict Outcomes

Focusing on a patient's symptoms is key to understanding lacrimal pathology, as patients will commonly describe one, or both, of 2 important symptom complexes.[3] The first group is volume symptoms, due to accumulation of debris in the lacrimal sac with backwash into the tear lake, and typically include recurrent bacterial conjunctivitis, dacryocystitis, episodic mucus regurgitation into the tear lake, and adherence of the eyelids on waking. The second symptom complex is flow symptoms and these arise due to the overall resistance of the lacrimal drainage pathway to tear flow. Such flow symptoms vary with the rate of tear production, but are usually associated with a welling-up of the tear lake, affecting vision and tear spillage from the eye.

When considering surgery for consenting patients, it is important to counsel patients according to their symptoms: volume symptoms (resulting from debris within the sac) can always be cured by DCR. In contrast, even if anatomically patent, some patients with a high tear production and/or relative resistance to canalicular flow (typically <10%) continue to have flow symptoms after DCR. A focus on symptomatology also concentrates the ophthalmologist in his or her understanding of the relationship between symptoms, underlying pathology, and surgical objectives.[4]

Canalicular Bypass Tubes

Lester Jones canalicular bypass tubes (LJTs) are the backbone of treatment for canalicular insufficiency. These large-bore flanged Pyrex glass tubes are positioned between the inner canthus and nasal cavity. Positioning of LJTs generally requires carunculectomy (but preserving the plica semilunaris) and should be inserted with adequate endonasal visualization to ensure clear placement within the nose. The tube should be angled downwards at 30 to 45 degrees in the coronal plane and emerge anterior to the middle turbinate. Episcleritis can occur if the ocular flange is posteriorly-directed and, if severe, this can lead to erosive scleritis.

Although LJTs provide symptomatic control to over 90% of patients, they have a low—but long-term—propensity to extrude[5] and various tube modifications have been proposed to reduce this risk. To improve grip and retention, LJTs have been designed with a midpoint bulge, surface frosting, a sheath of porous polythene, and, most recently, with a distal flange. Although the principle of these designs seems logical, the surface irregularity and larger area is associated with markedly increased accumulation of biofilm and a gross inflammatory response. The human surface tends to expel embedded foreign bodies (particularly in wet areas, where abundant organisms and mucus secretion accelerates biofilm formation) and all of these surface-modified tubes are liable to inflammatory extrusion or formation of pyogenic granulomas. Indeed, the key to a well-functioning LJT is the ability to easily remove and replace it as an outpatient, where regular cleaning—inside and outside—will remove any accumulated biofilm and prevent inflammatory extrusion of the device. Smooth-surfaced tubes should, therefore, be the device of choice in all cases. Our early experience of distally flanged tubes suggests that, while this design might aid retention, debris rapidly accumulates around the flange and tends to block the nasal end, leading to functional failure.

References

1. Gibbs DC. New probe for the intubation of lacrimal canaliculi with silicone rubber tubing. *Br J Ophthalmol.* 1967;51:198.
2. Chong KK, Lai FH, Ho M, Luk A, Wong BW, Young A. Randomized trial on silicone intubation in endoscopic mechanical dacryocystorhinostomy (SEND) for primary nasolacrimal duct obstruction. *Ophthalmology.* 2013;120:2139-2145.
3. Rose GE. The lacrimal paradox: toward a greater understanding of success in lacrimal surgery. *Ophthal Plast Reconstr Surg.* 2004;20:262-265.
4. Rose GE, Verity DH. Functional nasolacrimal duct obstruction: a nonexistent condition? Concepts in lacrimal dynamics and a practical course of treatment. *Expert Rev Ophthalmol.* 2011;6:603-610.
5. Rose GE, Welham RA. Jones' lacrimal canalicular bypass tubes: twenty-five years' experience. *Eye.* 1991;5:13-19.

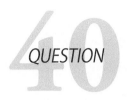

WHEN MANAGING PATIENTS WITH CONGENITAL NASOLACRIMAL DUCT OBSTRUCTION, DOES BALLOON DACRYOPLASTY WORK?

Jonathan Song, MD

Do you use balloon dacryoplasty? Does it really improve outcomes? Which patients should be offered balloon dacryoplasty?

Fortunately, most patients with congenital nasolacrimal duct obstruction (NLDO) do well with simple measures. When confronted with a child aged younger than 1 year with NLDO, my preferred management strategy is observation. I may suggest to some diligent parents to try gentle message over the lacrimal sac. Because the majority of patients improve spontaneously, I prefer to defer more invasive intervention until 1 year of age. When obstruction persists past 1 year of age, I usually recommend simple probing and irrigation. Rarely, if forced by infection or a symptomatic nasal mucocele, I may intervene at an age less than 1 year. In patients who fail probing and irrigation or who present at a later age (3 years or older), I consider more invasive therapy. Considerations include stenting and balloon dacryoplasty.

Balloon dacryoplasty refers to placing a probe that is surrounded by a water balloon into the nasolacrimal duct (Figure 40-1). The balloon is repeatedly inflated to fairly high pressures and then removed. For those comfortable with probing the nasolacrimal duct of children, the procedure is quite simple from a technical standpoint. The cost of the disposable equipment may be prohibitive in some cases. There are some variations in technique.

Technique

Select the size of catheter appropriate for your patient: 2 mm for patients younger than 30 months, 3 mm for patients 30 months and older. With the patient under general anesthesia, place a nasolacrimal duct probe through the nasolacrimal duct into the nose. Remove the probe. This confirms patency of the bony canal. Now pass the balloon catheter through nasolacrimal duct until its distal end is in the nose balloon. There are 2 markings on the proximal catheter shaft that

Kersten RC, McCulley TJ, eds. *Curbside Consultation in Oculoplastics:*
49 Clinical Questions, Second Edition (pp 205-207).
© 2016 Taylor & Francis Group.

Figure 40-1. The balloon catheter has been passed into the nasolacrimal duct. Note the black bars indicating the 15- and 10-mm distances from the proximal end of the balloon.

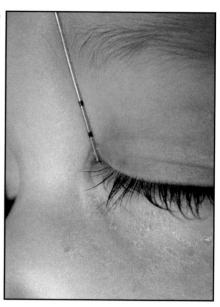

are 10 and 15 mm from the beginning of the working portion of the balloon. Pull the balloon proximally until the punctum is roughly aligned with the 15-mm mark. The balloon is gradually inflated to 8 atm for 90 seconds. Deflate the balloon. An additional inflation can be done (8 atm for 60 seconds) while aligned with the 10 mm mark. Deflate the balloon and withdraw the catheter.

Recommendations

Balloon dacryoplasty dilatation was first described as an alternative to simple intubation. It combines simple probing with mechanical dilation of the nasolacrimal duct with inflating and subsequently deflating a balloon that surrounds the distal stent. There's a fair amount of anecdotal support for its use. For example, Becker used this technique to treat 51 children older than 12 months (mean 26 months with 58% having had previous treatment failures) and reported success of 95%.[1] Similarly, Tao described overall 76.7% complete resolution of symptoms in children aged older than 18 months who have failed lacrimal probing or silicone intubation that underwent balloon catheter dilatation.[2] Studies such as these are always hard to interpret. There are a couple of controlled studies. Goldstein et al compared balloon dacryoplasty with monocanalicular intubation as secondary treatment of congenital nasolacrimal duct obstruction in children with failed probing. They reported success rates of 91% for monocanalicular intubation and 86% for balloon dacryoplasty. Further statistical analysis showed no significant difference between the 2 treatments or on the basis of age stratification within each treatment group.[3]

In one of the more carefully designed studies to date, the Pediatric Eye Disease Investigator Group (PEDIG) conducted a prospective, nonrandomized, multicenter study that enrolled 159 children aged 6 months to 48 months who had a history of a single failed nasolacrimal duct probing. Treatment success was reported to be 77% in the balloon catheter dilation group compared with 84% in the nasolacrimal intubation group.[4] In a second study, PEDIG also reported that balloon catheter dilation as a primary treatment of NLDO was successful in about 80% of cases in children aged 12 to 48 months. They noted that because they did not perform a randomized trial with a comparison group, they were unable to compare this procedure's success with that of simple probing or nasolacrimal intubation in this age group.[5]

Based on current studies, balloon dacryoplasty does work both as a primary or secondary procedure in the treatment of congenital nasal lacrimal duct obstruction. However, we don't know whether it is better than stenting, or how balloon dacryoplasty combined with stenting compares to stenting alone. My approach in patients with congenital NLDO who are aged younger than 2 years is simple probing, followed by stenting in failed cases. Based on cost and lack of proven effectiveness, I find that I rarely recommend balloon dacryoplasty and tend to reserve it for the more challenging cases in which the next step would be dacryocystorhinostomy.

References

1. Becker BB, Berry FD, Koller H. Balloon catheter dilatation for treatment of congenital nasolacrimal duct obstruction. *Am J Ophthalmol.* 1996;121:304-309.
2. Tao S, Meyer DR, Simon JW, Zobal-Ratner J. Success of balloon catheter dilatation as a primary or secondary procedure for congenital nasolacrimal duct obstruction. *Ophthalmology.* 2002;11:2108-2111.
3. Goldstein SM, Goldstein JB, Katowitz JA. Comparison of monocanalicular stenting and balloon dacryoplasty in secondary treatment of congenital nasolacrimal duct obstruction after failed primary probing. *Ophthal Plast Reconstr Surg.* 2004;20:352-357.
4. Repka MX, Chandler DL, Holmes JM, Pediatric Eye Disease Investigator Group. Balloon catheter dilation and nasolacrimal duct intubation for treatment of nasolacrimal duct obstruction after failed probing. *Arch Ophthalmol.* 2009;127:633-639.
5. Repka MX, Melia BM, Beck RW, Pediatric Eye Disease Investigator Group. Primary treatment of nasolacrimal duct obstruction with balloon catheter dilation in children younger than 4 years of age. *J AAPOS.* 2008;12(5):451-455.

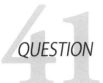

What Medications Cause Canalicular Obstruction and How Do You Prevent or Manage It?

Bita Esmaeli, MD, FACS

Is there an alternative to stenting? How do you evaluate patients with epiphora? Is canalicular obstruction the only way chemotherapeutic medications cause epiphora?

In cancer patients undergoing chemotherapy, excessive tearing is common. It is important to distinguish between excessive tearing, which is a symptom, and canalicular and nasolacrimal duct blockage, which are anatomic findings noted on probing and irrigation. Many chemotherapeutic drugs are associated with ocular surface irritation, conjunctivitis, tear film insufficiency, or blepharitis, all of which are known causes of pseudoepiphora. In contrast, to our knowledge, only 5 drugs, docetaxel (Taxotere), 5-fluorouracil (5-FU), S-1, iodine 131, and topical mitomycin C, have to date been fairly widely reported to cause blockage of the lacrimal outflow system.[1-23]

Chemotherapy Drugs That Cause Canalicular or Nasolacrimal Duct Blockage

Docetaxel

Docetaxel is a potent taxane used in the treatment of breast and prostate cancer and many other solid tumors.[24] A common adverse effect of docetaxel is canalicular stenosis.[1-4] Docetaxel is secreted in the tears, and this may be one mechanism by which docetaxel can cause canalicular inflammation with the end result of canalicular and nasolacrimal duct scarring and blockage.[4]

The schedule of administration of docetaxel influences the risk for lacrimal system blockage. In a prospective study, some colleagues and I reported that 64% of patients receiving weekly docetaxel

Kersten RC, McCulley TJ, eds. *Curbside Consultation in Oculoplastics: 49 Clinical Questions, Second Edition* (pp 209-214). © 2016 Taylor & Francis Group.

developed epiphora, in contrast to only about 39% of patients receiving docetaxel every 3 weeks.[3] We also found that one-third of the patients receiving weekly docetaxel developed moderate to severe canalicular blockage as an anatomic finding on probing and irrigation, whereas patients on the every 3 weeks schedule had epiphora but no evidence of canalicular blockage. This significant difference in frequency and severity of canalicular blockage with the 2 different schedules of administration of docetaxel is often not appreciated by oncologists or ophthalmologists. Despite numerous publications on this topic,[3-6] many oncologists and general ophthalmologists still do not appreciate the risk for permanent canalicular blockage in patients who are exposed to weekly administration of docetaxel and are at high risk for canalicular blockage. At the same time, some oculoplastic surgeons may prematurely subject a patient to unnecessary prophylactic silicone intubation, for example in patients who may be receiving every-3-weeks docetaxel for a short period of time, such as in the neoadjuvant setting.

5-Fluorouracil

A fluorinated pyrimidine used in the treatment of colon, breast, rectal, stomach, and pancreatic cancer, 5-FU can cause various degrees of mucosal inflammation, and it is thought to be secreted in the tear film, similar to docetaxel.[11] When 5-FU is administered intravenously, it is thought to be secreted by the lacrimal gland, causing ocular surface irritation and excessive tearing, which usually resolves following discontinuation of the drug.[8] Eiseman et al found that among 52 patients receiving intravenous 5-FU for at least 3 months, 14 patients (27%) developed excessive tearing, while only 4 (5.8%) had the anatomic correlative finding of punctal or canalicular stenosis.[9] Obstruction of the entire lacrimal drainage pathway, including the puncta, canaliculi, lacrimal sac, and duct, has been reported in patients receiving long-term therapy with 5-FU.[10] The risk for canalicular and nasolacrimal duct blockage is believed to be related to the total dose of drug and duration of treatment.[11]

Surgical intervention for patients with blockage of the lacrimal drainage apparatus due to 5-FU usually involves a dacryocystorhinostomy (DCR) with placement of silicone tubes; however, the degree of punctal and canalicular stenosis in the majority of patients treated with the modern dosing regimen of 5-FU is quite mild. Fezza et al reported that about one quarter of patients with 5-FU-induced nasolacrimal duct blockage required a conjunctivo-DCR and placement of a Pyrex glass tube because of the severity of canalicular scarring.[12] In my own practice at a tertiary cancer center where large numbers of patients with cancer are treated with the modern intravenous doses of 5-FU as a single agent or in combination with other chemotherapy drugs, cases of severe canalicular or nasolacrimal duct blockage are quite rare. This agent has also been associated with dermatitis, cicatricial ectropion, keratinization of the eyelid margin, madarosis, and ankyloblepharon.[13]

S-1

S-1 is an oral antineoplastic drug that is a 5-FU prodrug. It was designed with the idea that it might have fewer reported side effects than 5-FU. S-1 is approved in Japan for use in the treatment of gastrointestinal cancer, but it was not approved by the US Food and Drug Administration, perhaps because of genetic variations in the study populations in the two countries.[14]

S-1 was first reported to cause epiphora and severe canalicular stenosis in 2005 in an American patient who was being treated in a phase II study of S-1.[15] In a more recent study from Japan, 5 of 52 patients (9.6%) treated with S-1 experienced lacrimal stenosis. These investigators reported that 1 patient had punctal stenosis and 5 patients had canalicular stenosis. The time to onset of epiphora ranged from 2 to 8 months after the initiation of treatment with S-1.[16] The etiology of canalicular stenosis in patients receiving S-1 has not been studied; however, given that S-1 is a prodrug of 5-FU, the mechanism of S-1-induced canalicular stenosis may be similar to that of 5-FU-induced canalicular stenosis.

TOPICAL MITOMYCIN C

Punctal and canalicular stenosis have also been reported with topical mitomycin C.[17-19] A retrospective study of 100 eyes treated with topical mitomycin C (0.04%) 4 times a day for one to three 7-day cycles estimated about a 14% incidence of epiphora and punctal stenosis.[19]

RADIOACTIVE IODINE

Treatment of thyroid carcinoma with radioactive iodine, iodine 131 (^{131}I), has been reported to cause nasolacrimal duct obstruction with an estimated incidence of 3% to 4%.[20-22] The same iodine symporter found in the thyroid gland that is responsible for uptake of ^{131}I has also been found in the epithelium of the lacrimal sac and nasolacrimal duct but not in the canaliculi.[23] Thus, exposure to ^{131}I can cause inflammation and scarring of the lacrimal sac and nasolacrimal duct, resulting in nasolacrimal duct obstruction. Patients with nasolacrimal duct blockage associated with ^{131}I generally do well after a standard DCR and silicone tube placement; canalicular blockage is not as much of a problem. Silicone tubes may have to be left in place for the duration of anticipated treatment with ^{131}I.

Epiphora Associated With Other Chemotherapeutic Drugs

I have encountered temporary and mild epiphora in association with paclitaxel (Taxol), capecitabine (Xeloda), and imatinib mesylate (Gleevec), but have not observed significant punctal or canalicular stenosis associated with these drugs.

Paclitaxel (Taxol) is a taxane in the same family as docetaxel (Taxotere). I have personally evaluated many patients complaining of epiphora associated with paclitaxel, but to date, I have not observed anatomic closure of the puncta and canaliculi in association with the use of paclitaxel. There is one reported case of nasolacrimal duct blockage and canalicular stenosis in a patient who received paclitaxel,[25,26] but this patient also received head and neck radiation therapy, which is a well-known risk factor for canalicular stenosis and nasolacrimal duct blockage[27]; thus, it is difficult to attribute this single case of canalicular blockage and nasolacrimal duct blockage to exposure to paclitaxel.

Similarly, imatinib mesylate can be associated with the onset of epiphora in patients with chronic myelogenous leukemia or gastrointestinal stromal tumors who take this drug on a long-term basis. However, in our experience, the epiphora from imatinib is not associated with the anatomic findings of punctal and/or canalicular stenosis or nasolacrimal duct blockage.[28] Epiphora in patients chronically exposed to imatinib is most likely caused by fluid retention in the periorbital soft tissues and conjunctival chemosis, causing an inefficient blink and lacrimal pump.[29] Epiphora associated with imatinib can be treated in the majority of patients with nonsurgical measures such as the use of systemic diuretics or topical steroids.

Evaluation of Cancer Patients With Tearing

Evaluation of cancer patients with suspected nasolacrimal duct obstruction requires taking a thorough history with attention to symptoms and signs of epiphora, other ongoing medical problems, cancer history, medications used (including previous chemotherapy), radiation therapy, and surgeries in the orbitofacial area. Particular attention should be paid to the appearance and position of the lower eyelid and puncta, and it is important to carefully search for masses in the medial canthus, nose, and periorbital area. An abnormal skin texture, absence of a rash on the periocular skin, or blepharitis may be clues to causes of epiphora other than canalicular or nasolacrimal duct blockage. Probing and irrigation of the lacrimal drainage apparatus should be performed, and it should be noted whether there is any resistance in the canalicular system (a soft stop), how far a probe can be passed, and whether fluid refluxes out of or passes into the nasopharynx. A Schirmer's test can provide useful information about tear production, and although a Schirmer's test is not accurate in every patient, it can help identify dry eye syndrome, a common cause of pseudoepiphora.

Special tests such as the dye disappearance test, Jones I test, Jones II test, and lacrimal scintigraphy scans are less commonly used in daily practice but can be considered in selected patients in whom the diagnosis of canalicular or nasolacrimal blockage is in doubt.

Management of Canalicular and Nasolacrimal Duct Obstruction Associated With Chemotherapy

Epiphora in Patients Receiving Docetaxel Every 3 Weeks or for Short Periods

In the case of mild, early canalicular or nasolacrimal duct obstruction associated with chemotherapy, probing and irrigation followed by judicious use of topical steroid drops on a tapering dose may provide relief of epiphora. In the majority of patients with epiphora who are receiving docetaxel every 3 weeks or who will be exposed to docetaxel for a short period (less than 3 to 4 months), my preferred approach is frequent in-office probing and irrigation followed by topical steroid administration as appropriate and may be more than enough to relieve epiphora and prevent permanent blockage of canaliculi.[3-6,30,31] A perfect example would be patients who are receiving docetaxel as neoadjuvant or adjuvant therapy for breast cancer. A recent publication and associated editorial addressed the issues surrounding the management of epiphora in patients who are receiving docetaxel as adjuvant or neoadjuvant therapy and only for short periods.[32,33] In such patients, the risk for permanent canalicular blockage is quite low.

Epiphora in Patients Receiving Docetaxel Weekly or for Longer Duration

In patients who are receiving docetaxel weekly or in patients with metastatic disease for whom treatment duration is expected to be much longer, the risk for canalicular stenosis is much higher.[3,30,31] This risk is high enough to justify placement of silicone stents as soon as patients on weekly docetaxel develop epiphora and start to demonstrate progressive signs of punctal and canalicular blockage on probing and irrigation, such as pain, bleeding, or a soft stop on probing. When recurrent or progressive canalicular stenosis is observed on probing and irrigation, early bicanalicular silicone intubation should be strongly considered. Bicanalicular silicone intubation may prevent permanent canalicular blockage and the need for more invasive surgery such as DCR or conjunctivo-DCR.[6] The silicone tubes should be left in place for at least 2 to 3 months after cessation of docetaxel.[6]

Punctal Plugs and Monocanalicular Stents?

A commonly asked question is, "Why not use punctal plugs or monocanalicular stents that can be easily inserted in the office without anesthesia and might keep the puncta and canaliculi open?" The reason punctal plugs or monocanalicular stents are not the best choice for patients with epiphora associated with chemotherapy is that these devices block the tear drainage pathway and thus do not improve epiphora in patients who need to take a drug long term for metastatic disease. As noted previously, patients with metastatic disease likely will be exposed to docetaxel for long periods and are the only group of patients who are at high risk for canalicular blockage due to docetaxel. In such patients, insertion of a punctal plug or a monocanalicular stent will not relieve the debilitating symptom of epiphora. Furthermore, punctal plugs do not address the need to also protect the nasolacrimal duct and lacrimal sac from the inflammation and scarring that is known to also occur in the more distal portion of the nasolacrimal duct and nasal mucosa with both docetaxel and 5-FU.[4,10]

Anatomic Blockage of the Nasolacrimal Duct

For anatomic blockage of the nasolacrimal duct, DCR is the standard treatment. This procedure creates a connection between the lacrimal sac and the middle meatus of the nose, bypassing the nasolacrimal duct. Silicone stents are placed at the time of surgery to maintain patency during the first few months after surgery. Again, in the cases of combined canalicular and nasolacrimal duct blockage secondary to weekly docetaxel, the silicone stents should be left in for the duration of treatment with docetaxel and until at least 3 to 4 months after cessation of therapy.

DCR can be performed via an open external approach or via an endoscopic approach. Much debate exists over which method is preferable, but the debate between the advocates of external vs endoscopic DCR is outside the scope of this chapter. Both techniques have been widely used and reported in patients with idiopathic acquired nasolacrimal duct obstruction. Most studies report a higher failure rate with the endoscopic approach. In our practice, which mostly includes cancer patients with severe canalicular stenosis and abnormal anatomy due to prior surgery or other therapies, external DCR is preferred.

If the canaliculi are significantly obstructed, a conjunctivo-DCR with Pyrex glass tube (Jones tube) placement may become necessary and is the only option for symptomatic relief of epiphora. Complications are more common in patients requiring Jones tube placement than in patients undergoing a standard DCR. In a study of 49 patients who had Jones tube placement, extrusion, obstruction, and malposition were the most common complications, seen in 49%, 47%, and 33% of treated patients, respectively.[34] Other complications included discomfort, infection, and diplopia. Despite these known complications, 70% of patients who underwent a conjunctivo-DCR were satisfied after the procedure.

References

1. Esmaeli B, Valero V, Ahmadi MA, Booser D. Canalicular stenosis secondary to docetaxel (Taxotere): a newly recognized side effect. *Ophthalmology.* 2001;108(5):994-995.
2. Esmaeli B, Hidaji L, Adinin RB, et al. Blockage of the lacrimal drainage apparatus as a side effect of docetaxel therapy. *Cancer.* 2003;98(3):504-507.
3. Esmaeli B, Amin S, Valero V, et al. Prospective study of incidence and severity of epiphora and canalicular stenosis in patients with metastatic breast cancer receiving docetaxel. *J Clin Oncol.* 2006;24(22):3619-3622.

4. Esmaeli B, Burnstine MA, Ahmadi MA, Prieto VG. Docetaxel-induced histologic changes in the lacrimal sac and the nasal mucosa. *Ophthal Plast Reconstr Surg.* 2003;19(4):305-308.

5. Esmaeli B, Ahmadi MA, Rivera E, et al. Docetaxel secretion in tears: association with lacrimal drainage obstruction. *Arch Ophthalmol.* 2002;120(9):1180-1182.

6. Ahmadi MA, Esmaeli B. Surgical treatment of canalicular stenosis in patients receiving docetaxel weekly. *Arch Ophthalmol.* 2001;119(12):1802-1804.

7. Christophidis N, Vajda F, Lucas I, Louis W. Ocular side effects with 5-fluorouracil. *Aust N Z J Med.* 1979;9(2):143-144.

8. Prasad S, Kamath GG, Phillips RP. Lacrimal canalicular stenosis associated with systemic 5-fluorouracil therapy. *Acta Ophthalmol Scand.* 2000;78(1):110-113.

9. Eiseman AS, Flanagan JC, Brooks AB, Mitchell EP, Pemberton CH. Ocular surface, ocular adnexal, and lacrimal complications associated with the use of systemic 5-fluorouracil. *Ophthal Plast Reconstr Surg.* 2003;19(3):216-224.

10. Haidak DJ, Hurwitz BS, Yeung KY. Tear-duct fibrosis (dacryostenosis) due to 5-fluorouracil. *Ann Intern Med.* 1978;88(5):657.

11. Hassan A, Hurwitz J, Burkes R. Epiphora in patients receiving systemic 5-fluorouracil therapy. *Can J Ophthalmol.* 1998;33(1):14-19.

12. Fezza J, Wesley R, Klippenstein K. The treatment of punctal and canalicular stenosis in patients on systemic 5-FU. *Ophthalmic Surg Lasers.* 1999;30(2):105-108.

13. Ng J. Ocular side effects of cancer therapy. In: Esmaeli B, ed. *Ophthalmic Oncology.* Springer-Verlag; 2010:327-337.

14. Schoffski PA. The modulated oral fluoropyrimidine prodrug S-1, and its use in gastrointestinal cancer and other solid tumors. *Anticancer Drugs.* 2004;15(2):85-106.

15. Esmaeli B, Golio D, Lubecki L, Ajani J. Canalicular and nasolacrimal duct blockage: an ocular side effect associated with the antineoplastic drug S-1. *Am J Ophthalmol.* 2005;140(2):325-327.

16. Sasaki T, Miyashita H, Miyanaga T, et al. Dacryoendoscopic observation and incidence of canalicular obstruction/stenosis associated with S-1, an oral anticancer drug. *Jpn J Ophthalmol.* 2012;56:214-218.

17. Kopp E, Seregard S. Epiphora as a side effect of topical mitomycin C. *Br J Ophthalmol.* 2004;88(11):1422-1424.

18. Billing K, Karagiannis A, Selva D. Punctal-canalicular stenosis associated with mitomycin-C for corneal epithelial dysplasia. *Am J Ophthalmol.* 2003;136(4):746-747.

19. Khong JJ, Muecke J. Complications of mitomycin C therapy in 100 eyes with ocular surface neoplasia. *Br J Ophthalmol.* 2006;90(7):819-822.

20. Kloos R, Duvuuri V, Jhaing S, Cahill K, Foster J, Burns J. Nasolacrimal drainage system obstruction from radioactive iodine therapy for thyroid carcinoma. *J Clin Endocrinol Metab.* 2002;87:5817-5820.

21. Shepler T, Sherman S, Faustina M, Busaidy N, Ahmadi M, Esmaeli B. Nasolacrimal duct obstruction associated with radioactive iodine therapy for thyroid carcinoma. *Ophthal Plast Reconstr Surg.* 2003;19(6):479-481.

22. Burns J, Morgenstern K, Cahill K, Foster J, Jhiang S, Kloos R. Nasolacrimal obstruction secondary to I(131) therapy. *Ophthal Plast Reconstr Surg.* 2004;20(2):126-129.

23. Morgenstern K, Vadysirisack D, Zhang Z, et al. Expression of sodium iodide symporter in the lacrimal drainage system: implication for the mechanism underlying nasolacrimal duct obstruction in I(131)-treated patients. *Ophthal Plast Reconstr Surg.* 2005;21(5):337-344.

24. Valero V. Primary chemotherapy with docetaxel for the management of breast cancer. *Oncology.* 2002;16:35-43.

25. McCartney E, Valluri S, Rushing D, et al. Upper and lower system nasolacrimal duct stenosis secondary to paclitaxel. *Ophthal Plast Reconstr Surg.* 2007;23:170-171.

26. Savar A, Esmaeli B. Upper and lower system nasolacrimal duct stenosis secondary to paclitaxel. *Ophthal Plast Reconstr Surg.* 2009;25:418-419.

27. El-Sawy T, Ali R, Nasser QJ, Esmaeli B. Outcomes of dacryocystorhinostomy in patients with head and neck cancer treated with high-dose radiation therapy. *Ophthal Plast Reconstr Surg.* 2012;28(3):196-198.

28. Esmaeli B, Diba R, Ahmadi MA, et al. Periorbital edema and epiphora as ocular side effects of imatinib mesylate (Gleevec). *Eye.* 2004;18:760-762.

29. Esmaeli B, Prieto VG, Butler CE, et al. Severe periorbital edema secondary to STI571 (Gleevec). *Cancer.* 2002;95:881-887.

30. Saadati HG, Diba R, Esmaeli B. Lacrimal drainage blockage due to docetaxel. *Am J Oncology Rev.* 2003;2:608-611.

31. Esmaeli B. Management of excessive tearing as a side effect of docetaxel. *Clin Breast Cancer.* 2005;5:455-457.

32. Chan A, Su C, de Boer RH, et al. Prevalence of excessive tearing in women with early breast cancer receiving adjuvant docetaxel-based chemotherapy. *J Clin Oncol.* 2013;31:2123-2127.

33. Esmaeli B, Valero V. Epiphora and canalicular stenosis associated with adjuvant docetaxel in early breast cancer: is excessive tearing clinically important? *J Clin Oncol.* 2013;31(17):2076-2077.

34. Lim C, Martin P, Benger R, et al. Lacrimal canalicular bypass surgery with the Lester Jones tube. *Am J Ophthalmol.* 2004;137:101-108.

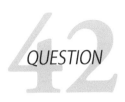

Is Anything New in the Management of Patients With Canalicular Obstruction?

Thomas E. Johnson, MD and
Sophie Liao, MD

What causes canalicular obstruction? Do all patients require surgery? What do you try before placing a Jones tube?

Canalicular obstruction is a fairly common cause of epiphora. It can occur in conjunction with and independent of nasolacrimal duct obstruction (NLDO). Observation comes with some risk for canaliculitis and further blockage, but may be indicated in asymptomatic patients, or those with dry eyes.

Most cases we see are acquired. In rare cases, congenital agenesis of the punctae and canaliculi may be the underlying etiology. Causative factors of acquired obstruction include the chronic use of a multitude of topical ocular medications (idoxuridine, echothiophate iodide, intraocular pressure-lowering eye drops, and antibiotics).[1] Other risk factors include chronic blepharitis, infectious canaliculitis, orbital radiation, trauma (accidental and surgical), retention of canalicular foreign bodies (punctual and canalicular plugs), and ocular surface diseases (Stevens-Johnson syndrome, ocular cicatricial pemphigoid, and herpetic disease).[2-6] Less commonly, neoplasms involving the medial eyelid may cause mechanical obstruction.

The use of certain systemic oncologic agents, most notably docetaxel and 5-fluorouracil (5-FU), is well documented to cause canalicular obstruction. With the advent of newer chemotherapeutic agents, canalicular stenosis as an adverse effect has been described in at least one newer anti-cancer agent, S-1, which is a combination of tegafur, 5-chloro-2, 4-dihydroxypyridine, and potassium oxonate, and is used for the treatment of colon, pancreatic, lung, and gastric cancer. The effects are possibly related to tegafur, which is a prodrug of 5-FU. 5-FU has been well described in other reports to be associated with canalicular fibrosis when administered systemically.[3,4,7] You can read more about this in Question 41.

Kersten RC, McCulley TJ, eds. *Curbside Consultation in Oculoplastics: 49 Clinical Questions, Second Edition* (pp 215-218).

Diagnosis may be made by a variety of methods. The fluorescein dye disappearance test, Jones I and II tests, and in-office punctal dilation, probing, and lacrimal irrigation are typically used in various combinations to localize a lacrimal drainage obstruction. Most often, all that is needed is probing and irrigation. Reflux of saline from the punctum being irrigated is indicative of canalicular obstruction; high-velocity reflux of saline from the opposite punctum indicates common canalicular obstruction. Office-based nasal endoscopy enables viewing of the nasal ostia and anatomy of the nasal turbinates and septum, which allows one to determine whether any nasal abnormality is a contributing factor. A newer instrument, the dacryoendoscope, is thinner than the traditional endoscope, and enables direct visualization of the canaliculi and localization of any obstruction. Sasaki et al described the use of this technology along with microscissors to directly visualize and excise common canalicular obstructions.[8]

Conjunctivodacryocystorhinostomy (CDCR), the creation of a fistula between the conjunctiva and nasal cavity, along with permanent placement of a Pyrex glass tube to keep the fistula open, has been considered the gold standard for treatment of canalicular obstruction or agenesis. Because patients may have difficulties with the presence of this permanent tube, including extrusion, migration, clogging, or discomfort from inhaled air or mucus reflux affecting the ocular surface, practitioners have sought to develop alternative methods of management. If the obstruction is localized in the bilateral distal canaliculi, with intact proximal canaliculi, a canaliculodacryocystorhinostomy may be performed with intubation. In this technique, the focal obstruction is excised through a standard DCR incision with anastomosis of the resulting canalicular ends to remaining lacrimal sac or nasal mucosa. Serial dilation of stenotic canaliculi, sharp probing, or direct excision of milder obstructions, followed by silicone stent intubation, may also be attempted. These less invasive methods are generally limited to more focal obstructions.[9] Recently, alternative surgical techniques have been described, including retrograde dacryoendoscopy with obstruction excision from a nasal approach, balloon canaliculoplasty, and canalicular trephination with or without the assistance of endoscopy.

Lacrimal trephination was first espoused by Sisler in the 1990s and has gained some traction. The mini-trephine is a 0.81-mm stainless steel tube fitted with a spring-assisted plunger and intraluminal stylet that allows for sharp excision of an intracanalicular obstruction under local anesthesia.[10] It has been reported to have variable success rates: Nathoo et al reported 83% functional and 84% anatomic success at 5.6 months. At 12 months, 16 of 45 trephinated patients remained patent and the other 29 patients required a second procedure; the success rate of reoperated patients was not reported separately.[11] Khoubian et al reported 49% of patients had complete relief, with an additional 38% of patients achieving partial relief of epiphora when trephination was combined with silicone intubation in cases of complete canalicular obstruction. They noted that patients with distal monocanalicular obstructions had the highest success rate, followed by distal bicanalicular, common canalicular, and proximal obstructions.[12]

Endoscopic DCR may be modified to include canalicular marsupialization for common canalicular obstruction (CCO). A routine endoscopic DCR is performed, with the addition of a slit-knife incision of the area of CCO, followed by placement of stents. Kim et al describe 81.6% success after a single procedure in 36 patients. Five additional patients had symptomatic relief of epiphora after a revision procedure for recurrent CCO or obstruction along the DCR tract. Presence of a distal canalicular obstruction was cited as a reason for failure.[13]

Balloon canaliculoplasty for stenotic, but not completely obstructed, canaliculi has been described with varying success rates. In this technique, a 2-mm balloon catheter is threaded through the entire canalicular length and inflated several times to manually dilate the lumen. Zoumalan et al reported success in 76.2% of patients treated in conjunction with silicone intubation, with a short follow-up time of 6 months.[14] Yang et al reported a 53.6% success rate in CCO patients, but only a 25% success rate in patients with monocanalicular obstruction at

12 months postprocedure when combining balloon canaliculoplasty with manual trephination and silicone intubation.[15]

Consideration should be given to prophylactic canalicular intubation in patients who will be on extended or frequent treatment with docetaxel, S-1, or 5-FU, given the association of these chemotherapeutic agents with canalicular fibrosis. Some investigators found that patients on weekly or prolonged therapy with docetaxel were more likely to develop canalicular obstructions compared to those on therapy administered once every 3 weeks, and those patients on a more intensive medication regimen were more likely to benefit from prophylactic stent placement.[16]

Summary

Canalicular obstruction should usually be identified and treated to avoid symptomatic epiphora and possible infection. If there is concomitant punctal or nasolacrimal stenosis, or osteomeatal disease, this should be treated simultaneously. Focal canalicular stenosis may be treated by attempted dilation, sharp probing, and intubation, or direct excision of the obstruction with reanastomosis with or without intubation. In more distal obstructions, lacrimal trephination techniques have been successful. If the canaliculi are stenotic but not completely obstructed, balloon canaliculoplasty may be useful. Severe distal, common canalicular, or complete bicanalicular obstruction may require treatment with a CDCR with a Jones tube or canaliculodacryocystorhinostomy with silicone stent intubation, although newer techniques of retrograde endo-DCR or dacryoendoscopic-assisted excision of canalicular obstructions have shown some promise.

References

1. McNab AA. Lacrimal canalicular obstruction associated with topical ocular medication. *Aust N Z J ophthalmol.* 1998;26(3):219-223.
2. Sanke RF, Welham RA. Lacrimal canalicular obstruction following chickenpox. *Br J Ophthalmol.* 1982;66(1):71-74.
3. Esmaeli B, Golio D, Lubecki L, Ajani J. Canalicular and nasolacrimal duct blockage: an ocular side effect associated with the antineoplastic drug S-1. *Am J Ophthalmol.* 2005;140(2):325-327.
4. Fezza JP, Wesley RE, Klippenstein KA. The treatment of punctal and canalicular stenosis in patients on systemic 5-FU. *Ophthalmic Surg Lasers.* 1999;30(2):105-108.
5. Haidak DJ, Hurwitz BS, Yeung KY. Tear-duct fibrosis (dacryostenosis) due to 5-fluorouracil. *Ann Intern Med.* 1978;88(5):657.
6. Harris GJ, Hyndiuk RA, Fox MJ, Taugher PJ. Herpetic canalicular obstruction. *Arch Ophthalmol.* 1981;99(2):282-283.
7. Sasaki T, Miyashita H, Miyanaga T, Yamamoto K, Sugiyama K. Dacryoendoscopic observation and incidence of canalicular obstruction/stenosis associated with S-1, an oral anticancer drug. *Jpn J Ophthalmol.* 2012;56(3):214-218.
8. Sasaki T, Sounou T, Sugiyama K. Dacryoendoscopic surgery and tube insertion in patients with common canalicular obstruction and ductal stenosis as a frequent complication. *Jpn J Ophthalmol.* 2009;53(2):145-150.
9. Tabatabaie SZ, Rajabi MT, Rajabi MB, Eshraghi B. Randomized study comparing the efficacy of a self-retaining bicanaliculus intubation stent with Crawford intubation in patients with canalicular obstruction. *Clin Ophthalmol.* 2012;6:5-8.
10. Sisler HA, Allarakhia L. New minitrephine makes lacrimal canalicular rehabilitation an office procedure. *Ophthal Plastic Reconstr Surg.* 1990;6(3):203-206.
11. Nathoo NA, Rath S, Wan D, Buffam F. Trephination for canalicular obstruction: experience in 45 eyes. *Orbit.* 2013;32(5):281-284.
12. Khoubian JF, Kikkawa DO, Gonnering RS. Trephination and silicone stent intubation for the treatment of canalicular obstruction: effect of the level of obstruction. *Ophthal Plastic Reconstr Surg.* 2006;22(4):248-252.
13. Kim DW, Choi MY, Shim WS. Endoscopic dacryocystorhinostomy with canalicular marsupialization in common canalicular obstruction. *Can J Ophthalmol.* 2013;48(4):335-339.

14. Zoumalan CI, Maher EA, Lelli GJ Jr, Lisman RD. Balloon canaliculoplasty for acquired canalicular stenosis. *Ophthal Plastic Reconstr Surg*. 2010;26(6):459-461.
15. Yang SW, Park HY, Kikkawa DO. Ballooning canaliculoplasty after lacrimal trephination in monocanalicular and common canalicular obstruction. *Jpn J Ophthalmol*. 2008;52(6):444-449.
16. Esmaeli B, Amin S, Valero V, et al. Prospective study of incidence and severity of epiphora and canalicular stenosis in patients with metastatic breast cancer receiving docetaxel. *J Clin Oncol*. 2006;24(22):3619-3622.

SECTION VI

MISCELLANEOUS

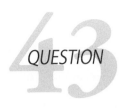

QUESTION

43

WHAT ROLE CAN ENDOSCOPES PLAY IN OCULOPLASTIC SURGERY?

Don O. Kikkawa, MD and
Jane S. Kim, MD

Do you use endoscopy in your practice? For which procedures do you find that it is most helpful?

Endoscopes are playing an increasingly important role in oculoplastic surgery and it is essential that every oculoplastic surgeon be familiar with their use. The requirements for implementation are an endoscope, adequate lighting, an optical cavity, and an imaging system with a camera. Endoscopes come in varying sizes and viewing angles, and each has differing indications for use. Since first being described in the early 1980s for foreign body removal,[1] endoscopes have found their role in lacrimal surgery,[2,3] aesthetic surgery,[4] orbital surgery,[5-7] and teaching.

Learning to use the endoscope does take some adjustment. The surgeon must look at a two-dimensional view on a monitor (Figure 43-1), while placing instruments in a three-dimensional field. Additionally, hemostasis must be optimal as even small amounts of bleeding may obscure the field. We find that the 30-degree, 4-mm endoscope (Figure 43-2) is the most versatile and can be used in lacrimal, orbital, and facial surgery.

Lacrimal surgery has the most widespread use of endoscopes. All types of lacrimal procedures can be performed with the endoscope, including dacryocystorhinostomy (primary and revision), conjunctival dacryocystorhinostomy with Jones tube placement, and congenital dacryocele management with intranasal extension. Although endonasal dacryocystorhinostomy has been described without the use of the endoscope, we find that endoscopic viewing offers several advantages. First, it offers fine detailed views of the lacrimal sac and common canaliculus. Second, it allows the surgeon to perform the osteotomy with finer control, being able to examine the exact location and relationship to important structures (Figure 43-3), including the middle turbinate, middle meatus, and uncinate process. Concurrent septoplasty may be performed if necessary. Finally, office examination with the endoscope allows the ability to preoperatively diagnose septal deviation and allergic rhinitis, rule out other intranasal pathology, and directly examine and debride the ostium postoperatively.

Kersten RC, McCulley TJ, eds. *Curbside Consultation in Oculoplastics:*
49 Clinical Questions, Second Edition (pp 221-224).
© 2016 Taylor & Francis Group.

Figure 43-1. Endoscopic tower and surgeon's view during endoscopic dacryocystorhinostomy.

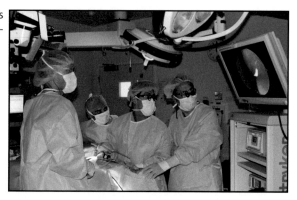

Figure 43-2. Thirty-degree 4-mm endoscope, one of the more versatile types of endoscopes used in orbital, oculofacial, and lacrimal surgery.

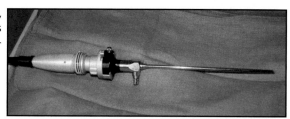

Figure 43-3. Left intranasal view with endoscope (NS=nasal septum, MT=middle turbinate, NL=location of nasolacrimal sac).

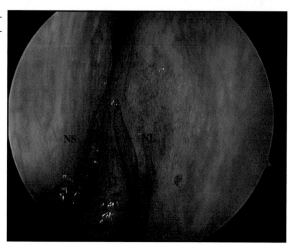

Aesthetic facial surgery is the next major area of use. Small-incision brow lifting and midface lifting have been revolutionized with the endoscope. Through limited scalp incisions, optical cavities can be created in the central forehead region and temporal regions. Under direct visualization within the optical cavities, vital facial structures can be avoided. For brow lifting, this includes the supraorbital neurovascular bundle (Figure 43-4) and the medial zygomatic temporal (sentinel) vein (Figure 43-5). During midface lifting, the infraorbital nerve, levator labii superioris, and zygomaticofacial nerve can be identified and preserved. Conservative myectomy of the corrugator supraciliaris and procerus can also be performed.

Endoscopic orbital surgery is the final frontier. The paranasal sinuses provide the perfect anatomic adjunct to create a combined sino-orbital optical cavity. The most common indication is endoscopic orbital decompression of the medial orbital wall and orbital floor for thyroid related orbitopathy. This is done in conjunction with endoscopic ethmoidectomy and sphenoidotomy.

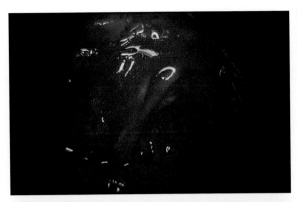

Figure 43-4. Endoscopic view of supraorbital nerve (arrow) during endoscopic forehead lifting.

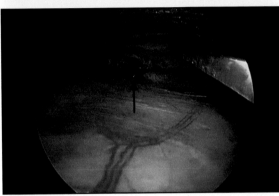

Figure 43-5. Endoscopic view of deep temporal vein (arrow) during endoscopic forehead lifting.

Medial periorbital incisions under direct endoscopic visualization allow the precise ability to preserve support adjacent to the medial and inferior rectus muscles and theoretically lessen muscle prolapse into the sinus cavities, lowering diplopia risk. With creation of a sino-orbital optical cavity, a variety of orbital apex masses can be removed, and image guidance offers additional precision. Furthermore, access to the sphenoid sinus allows visualization of the optic canal, which can be decompressed in the rare instance indicated in the treatment of indirect optic neuropathy. While not common indications, endoscopic orbital floor fracture[6] and intracranial approaches to the skull base are becoming more widely employed.[7]

Finally, we find the endoscope to be a great adjunct in teaching. Endoscopes are most useful for seeing things in tight spaces and visualizing things not easily seen. With orbital surgery, typically only the surgeon is able to visualize in the deep orbit. This creates difficulty in teaching orbital apex surgery. For educational video production, we routinely use the endoscope to capture operations that were heretofore only seen by the primary surgeon. This adjunct use has brought surgical instruction to a higher level.

Summary

Endoscopes serve an essential function in the surgical repertoire of the oculoplastic surgeon. Additional future indications will only further emphasize the importance of their role in modern oculofacial plastic and orbital surgery.

References

1. Norris JL. Endoscopic orbital surgery: report of a case. *Arch Ophthalmol.* 1981;99(8):1400-1401.
2. Watkins LM, Janfaza P, Rubin PA. The evolution of endonasal dacryocystorhinostomy. *Surv Ophthalmol.* 2003;48(1):73-84.
3. Hodgson N, Bratton E, Whipple K, et al. Outcomes of endonasal dacryocystorhinostomy without mucosal flap preservation. *Ophthal Plast Reconstr Surg.* 2014;30(1):24-27.
4. Hutcherson R, Keller GS. Endoscopic techniques in facial rejuvenation surgery. *Facial Plast Surg.* 1996;12(3):303-310.
5. Kennedy DW, Goodstein ML, Miller NR, Zinreich SJ. Endoscopic transnasal orbital decompression. *Arch Otolaryngol Head Neck Surg.* 1990;116(3):275-282.
6. Ducic Y, Verret DJ. Endoscopic transantral repair of orbital floor fractures. *Otolaryngol Head Neck Surg.* 2009;140(6):849-854.
7. Schaberg M, Murchison AP, Rosen MR, Evans JJ, Bilyk JR. Transorbital and transnasal endoscopic repair of a meningoencephalocele. *Orbit.* 2011;30(5):221-225.

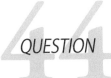

WHAT ARE AMERICAN COLLEGE OF CHEST PHYSICIANS RECOMMENDATIONS FOR MANAGEMENT OF ANTITHROMBOTIC THERAPY (ANTICOAGULATION) PERIOPERATIVELY AND ARE THEY APPLICABLE TO OCULOPLASTIC SURGERY?

Nicholas R. Mahoney, MD

What oculoplastic procedures are most at risk for complications related to bleeding? When needed, how long before surgery should I ask patients to stop taking their mediations? When should they restart them after surgery?

Significant perioperative bleeding can result in a variety of suboptimal outcomes in oculoplastic surgery. Some problems, such as unsightly facial bruising or epistaxis, are usually of limited consequence. Others, such as flap necrosis or graft failure, may result in a need for reoperation. The most catastrophic and feared complication from bleeding, a retrobulbar hemorrhage with resultant orbital compartment syndrome, can lead to permanent vision loss.[1] Antiplatelet and anticoagulant therapies are known risk factors for increased perioperative bleeding and, as such, the surgeon should be aware of their use. Medications that may increase bleeding used as needed for pain, such as nonsteroidal anti-inflammatories and aspirin, are often held preoperatively to decrease risk. Discontinuing medications prescribed for cardiovascular health, however, may increase systemic risk for coronary syndromes and stroke. Ultimately, the decision to stop antithrombotic therapy perioperatively should be individualized and must balance the risk and sequelae of adverse cardiovascular events and thromboembolism against those of perioperative bleeding.

Risk for Intraoperative Bleeding

The oculoplastic procedures often considered at higher risk for bleeding are those involving the nasolacrimal system, orbit, or skin flaps and/or grafts, but no specific studies for these procedures reporting on bleeding complication rates exist.[2] Blepharoplasty, which is the most common surgery in most oculoplastic surgery practices, often involves the postseptal orbital fat and has

Kersten RC, McCulley TJ, eds. *Curbside Consultation in Oculoplastics:*
49 Clinical Questions, Second Edition (pp 225-229).
© 2016 Taylor & Francis Group.

been studied regarding bleeding complications. The risk for retrobulbar hemorrhage after blepharoplasty was estimated to be 0.05% in a survey of American Society of Ophthalmic Plastic and Reconstructive Surgery members representing more than 250,000 patients.[3] About 8% of these patients suffered permanent vision loss and 26% of these patients were on aspirin.[3] A similar survey of plastic surgeons representing over 750,000 patients reported retrobulbar hemorrhage as the etiology in half of 0.0052% of patients with vision loss and reported 15% incidence of aspirin use.[1] It has been estimated that overall there is a 35% incidence of aspirin use in patients undergoing any oculoplastic surgery procedure.[4] These surveys do not suggest an increase in aspirin use in patients with bleeding complications and clearly indicate vision loss is rare. When retrobulbar hemorrhage occurs, it develops within the first 24 hours and presents uniformly with pain and occasionally with nausea or vision loss, and often requires immediate medical or surgical intervention.[3]

Although often discussed, there is also no conclusive evidence to prove an increased risk for poor outcomes in patients on antithrombotic therapies with the majority of intraocular ophthalmic procedures in general (a possible exception to this is warfarin use during trabeculotomy).[2] A meta-analysis reviewing the effects of anticoagulation on dermatologic procedures in prior retrospective studies representing 1373 patients found a 1.3% risk for severe bleeding in patients on antiplatelet therapy and 5.7% risk for severe bleeding in patients on warfarin compared to 0.5% risk in controls.[5] Unfortunately, the risk for cardiovascular events while withholding medications and the consequences of severe bleeding were not reported. In a retrospective review of 1015 oculoplastic surgery patients, Kent and Custer actually found a statistically significant decrease in bleeding risks in patients who continued their antiplatelet therapy compared to those who held it.[4]

The American College of Chest Physicians (ACCP) does recognize that an increased risk for bleeding exists in patients on antithrombotic therapy during "major surgery with extensive tissue injury, eg, reconstructive plastic surgery" as well as urologic surgery; pacemaker implantation; bowel, kidney, liver, and spleen surgery; and cardiac, intracranial and some spinal procedures.[6] Their guidelines, however, do not provide specific recommendations for continuing or withholding medications based on individual procedures or surgical specialties. The guidelines do make specific recommendations in the subcategories of minor dermatologic procedures and cataract surgery, where withholding antithrombotic therapy is not recommended based on the rarity of complications and unclear increase in risk in outcome based on anticoagulant use. As is discussed below, they recommend an assessment of the risk of bleeding and medication withholding and also provide strategies to discontinuing medications.

Antithrombotic Therapies

Antithrombotic medical therapies include both antiplatelet and anticoagulation medications. Aspirin and warfarin have been the most widely available and studied drugs of these categories, respectively, but new medications are emerging.

Antiplatelet Therapies

- Aspirin: cyclo-oxygenase 1 inactivation and inhibition of thromboxane production[2]
- Clopidogrel (Plavix)/Prasugrel (Effient): irreversible platelet P2Y12 receptor inhibitors[2]
- Ticagrelor (Brilinta)/Cangrelor (investigative): reversible P2Y12 antagonist[2]
- Dipyrdiamole (Persantine, Aggrenox with aspirin): reversible platelet aggregation inhibitor[2]

Anticoagulative Therapies

- Vitamin K antagonists: Warfarin(Coumadin), Acenocoumarol, Phenprocoumon, Anisindione: clotting factors II, VII, IX, and X inhibitors[2]
- Unfractionated and low molecular weight heparin: anti-thrombin activators[2]
- Apixaban (Eliquis)/Rivaroxaban (Xarelto): factor Xa inhibitors[2]
- Dabigatran (Pradaxa): thrombin inhibitor[2]

Other drugs that may influence thrombosis include nonsteroidal anti-inflammatory medications and several herbs including feverfew, garlic, ginger, ginkgo, and ginseng.[2] Vitamin E has an antithrombotic effect in the laboratory that has not been verified in humans.[4]

Indications for Antithrombotic Therapy

The two broad indications for antithrombotic use are primary and secondary prevention of cardiovascular and thromboembolic events. Low-dose aspirin antiplatelet therapy for the primary prevention of cardiovascular disease is currently recommended where there is no prior history of cardiovascular disease and no contraindication (eg, gastrointestinal bleeding) in:

- Nondiabetic men aged between 49 to 75 years
- Nondiabetic women aged between 55 to 75 years
- Diabetic men aged older than 50 years
- Diabetic women aged older than 60 years[6]

Daily aspirin use is also recommended for secondary prevention after coronary artery bypass grafting or in patients with a history of acute coronary syndrome.[6] Dual antiplatelet therapy, such as with daily aspirin and clopidogrel, is recommended for patients with a history of a cardiovascular stent. As mentioned, patients meeting criteria for antiplatelet use has been reported to account for 35% of oculoplastic surgical patients.[4] Despite this, in their review of oculoplastic surgery patients, Kent and Custer found 59% of patients who met criteria for daily aspirin use not on appropriate therapy.[4] In addition, they noted that 12% of patients on therapy neglected to disclose their aspirin use.[4]

Anticoagulation therapy is recommended for patients at high, moderate, and low risks for thromboembolic events. This risk is stratified by the ACCP on the basis of events observed in trials comparing patients on anticoagulant therapies to those on no therapy. In general, this stratification ignores risk to thromboembolism from the surgery itself and is an indirect inference from studies performed outside of the perioperative period. The 3 main indications for anticoagulative therapy are accounted for: a history of mechanical heart valve placement, atrial fibrillation, or prior venous thromboembolic events. Atrial fibrillation is accounted for using the CHADS2 scoring system (ie, a score based on history of congestive heart failure, hypertension, age, diabetes, and stroke). A high-risk patient has a >10% risk per year of an event and specific examples include a patient with a mitral valve prosthesis, rheumatic valvular heart disease, thromboembolism/stroke within the last 3 months, severe thrombophilia, or CHADS2 score of 5 or 6. A low-risk patient has <1% per year risk for an event and examples include patients with a bileaflet aortic valve prosthesis without atrial fibrillation, a CHADS2 score of 0 to 2, or a venous thromboembolism >1 year ago. A moderate-risk patient falls in the middle with regard to thromboembolism history or CHADS2 score.

Stopping Anticoagulants

When stopping therapy, the ACCP recommends withholding warfarin >5 days before surgery based on the half-life of 36 to 42 hours of the drug and retrospective studies demonstrating a return to international normalized ratio (INR) <1.5 in >90% of patients at this time. They recommend INR testing on the day before surgery when feasible and resumption of therapy the evening of surgery.[6] Bridging therapy (ie, conversion from a long- to a short-acting anticoagulant agent preoperatively) is recommended if warfarin is held in high-risk patients and recommended against if warfarin is held in low-risk patients. Moderate-risk patient decisions should be individualized, and the bridging itself can be accomplished with several regimens (essentially high-, intermediate-, or low-dose heparin therapy).[7] The ACCP does not specifically recommend one regimen, but unfractionated IV heparin is clearly less cost effective but similarly efficacious to subcutaneous low-molecular-weight heparin.[7] If unfractionated heparin is used, it should be stopped 4 to 6 hours before surgery.[7] Low-molecular-weight heparin should be stopped 24 hours before surgery and resumed 24 hours after surgery in non–high-bleeding-risk surgery such as most oculoplastic procedures.[7] If needed, reversal of warfarin can be achieved with intravenous vitamin K and fresh frozen plasma or prothrombin complex concentrate.[2] The timing of withholding other anticoagulants is not clearly established, but preliminary studies suggest rivaroxaban should be stopped at least 24 hours prior and apibaxan between 24 to 48 hours prior to surgery. Withholding diabigatran requires an assessment of the patient's renal function.[2]

Stopping Antiplatelet Agents

Patients receiving aspirin for primary prevention and at a moderate to high risk for cardiovascular adverse events include those with a history of ischemic heart disease, congestive heart failure, diabetes, renal insufficiency, and cerebrovascular disease. The ACCP recommends continuing acetylsalicylic acid (ASA) in these patients (surgery unspecified) based on meta-analyses of retrospective data representing 45,000 patients where a protective effect against cardiovascular events was noted without an increased risk for bleeding related reoperations. Low-risk patients, however, should stop therapy aspirin 7 to 10 days preoperatively.[7]

In patients receiving antiplatelet therapy for secondary prevention undergoing cataract or dermatologic surgery, the ACCP recommends continuing therapy,[7] which should likely be extended to a similar recommendation for most oculoplastic surgery.

Retrospective data regarding adverse events in patients on therapy after receiving stents suggest that patients on dual antiplatelet therapy should defer elective surgery for 6 weeks after bare-metal stent placement and 6 months after drug-eluting stent placement. In urgent cases, dual antiplatelet therapy should be continued.[7]

Most platelet inhibitors are essentially irreversible and therefore their duration of effect after cessation is irrespective of their half-life. Dipyridamole is reversible but is often administered with aspirin (Aggrenox). Common nonsteroidal anti-inflammatory medication half-lives range from short (2 to 6 hours for ibuprofen) to long (7 to 14 hours for naproxen). Aspirin's antiplatelet effect occurs within minutes, while clopidogrel takes 5 to 10 days unless a loading dose is used.[7] When aspirin is stopped, a rebound prothrombotic state may transiently occur.[4] In high-risk patients with both high risk for thromboembolic or adverse cardiovascular event and high risk of bleeding with potential for devastating outcomes, elective surgeries may need to be avoided.[4]

References

1. Mejia JD, Egro FM, Nahai F. Visual loss after blepharoplasty: incidence, management, and preventive measures. *Aesthet Surg J*. 2011;31:21-29.
2. Kiire CA, Mukherjee R, Ruparelia N, Keeling D, Prendergast B, Norris JH. Managing antiplatelet and anticoagulant drugs in patients undergoing elective ophthalmic surgery. *Br J Ophthalmol*. 2014;98(10):1320-1324.
3. Hass AN, Penne RB, Stefanyszyn MA, Flanagan JC. Incidence of postblepharoplasty orbital hemorrhage and associated visual loss. *Ophthal Plastic Reconstr Surg*. 2004;20:426-432.
4. Kent TL, Custer PL. Bleeding complications in both anticoagulated and nonanticoagulated surgical patients. *Ophthal Plastic Reconstr Surg*. 2013;29:113-117.
5. Lewis KG, Dufresne RG, Jr. A meta-analysis of complications attributed to anticoagulation among patients following cutaneous surgery. *Dermatol Surg*. 2008;34:160-164; discussion 4-5.
6. US Preventive Services Task Force. Aspirin for the prevention of cardiovascular disease: U.S. Preventive Services Task Force recommendation statement. *Ann Intern Med*. 2009;150(6):396-404.
7. Douketis JD, Spyropoulos AC, Spencer FA, et al. Perioperative management of antithrombotic therapy: Antithrombotic Therapy and Prevention of Thrombosis, 9th ed: American College of Chest Physicians Evidence-Based Clinical Practice Guidelines. *Chest*. 2012;141:e326S-350S.

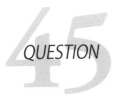

How Do I Decide Whether to Perform an Evisceration or Enucleation?

Thomas N. Hwang, MD, PhD

Do you prefer evisceration or enucleation? Are there specific situations where one is preferable? Which do you most often recommend?

As you know, both evisceration and enucleation result in replacement of the eye with a spherical artificial orbital implant. An evisceration involves completely removing the internal ocular contents and then separately closing the remaining scleral shell, Tenon's capsule, and conjunctiva over the implant. An enucleation involves removal of the entire globe along with a section of the optic nerve. The implant is then placed into the orbital fat. Often, the recti muscles are drawn forward and secured anteriorly, followed by separate closure of Tenon's capsule and conjunctiva.

Common indications for either technique include a ruptured globe as prophylaxis against sympathetic ophthalmia; a "blind, painful eye"; end-stage endophthalmitis; or a malignant intraocular tumor (most commonly a choroidal melanoma). A 1996 survey of the American Society of Ophthalmic Plastic and Reconstructive Surgery (ASOPRS) showed that enucleations were several times more common than eviscerations.[1] However, a more recent 2012 publication of an online survey of ASOPRS members showed that for cases not involving malignancy, evisceration is gaining popularity, especially among the more recently trained, with slightly over 60% preferring evisceration compared to slightly over 30% preferring enucleation and a small percentage having no preference.[2]

The issues involved in deciding whether to perform an evisceration or an enucleation fall into two categories—technical and medical. The technical aspects include orbital implant motility, resistance to extrusion, and size. The medical aspects include quality of pathologic specimen, containment of intraocular infection, clear removal of intraocular malignancy, and relationship to sympathetic ophthalmia.

In terms of motility, because the extraocular muscles remain attached to the sclera closed around the implant in an evisceration, the technique naturally provides excellent implant motility. In contrast, in a simplified enucleation, the recti muscles are allowed to fall back into the orbit,

Kersten RC, McCulley TJ, eds. *Curbside Consultation in Oculoplastics: 49 Clinical Questions, Second Edition* (pp 231-234).
© 2016 Taylor & Francis Group.

where they will eventually fuse with the capsule that forms around the implant. The implant will still move, but the muscles have a decreased mechanical advantage. Consequently, most surgeons tie off the 4 recti muscles before detaching them from the globe so that they can be drawn forward and tied anteriorly to the implant, directly to the implant, or to an artificial wrapping (like donor sclera) around the implant to provide better motility. For resistance to extrusion, the scleral closure in evisceration adds another complete layer of protection against implant extrusion. Both procedures have good success in terms of long-term stability. The key element in both procedures hinges on careful closure of each layer without tension.

Implant size has traditionally been considered a primary limitation of evisceration. A small implant size affects the ultimate cosmesis of the surgery because of the lack of orbital volume replacement. However, this limitation with evisceration has been largely overcome by a variety of scleral modification techniques that effectively allow the placement of larger implants. These techniques simply create an opening in the sclera large enough for the implant to pass into the orbital fat before closure so that the sclera does not limit the implant size.[3] Obviously, enucleation allows for easy placement of large implants.

As a concluding remark about the technical aspects, most of the above issues are relative issues. Most surgeons have a personal preference, and a skilled surgeon doing either technique will produce a good surgical result, although evisceration is arguably simpler and less invasive. Interestingly, based on a survey of ocularists who take care of these patients long term, eviscerations were preferred overwhelmingly over enucleations because of perceived superiority in cosmesis, motility, and lack of complications.[4]

From a medical standpoint, certain cases create an advantage of one procedure over the other. For example, a good pathologic specimen may be important to make a diagnosis. For this purpose, enucleation provides the ultimate gross and microscopic specimen because the globe is removed intact. Evisceration only allows for a disorganized collection of intraocular contents. Another common scenario involves cases of end-stage infectious endophthalmitis, when the eye is irreparable and becomes a pseudo-abscess. Evisceration likely provides a barrier that prevents infection from traveling. With an enucleation, the cut optic nerve may provide a conduit for microorganisms via the subarachnoid space.

The one dogma that does exist when considering enucleation or evisceration is the absolute contraindication to evisceration with a known intraocular malignancy, most commonly a choroidal melanoma. In this case, clearly the risk for microscopic seeding of the orbit during an evisceration is unacceptable. However, the more unclear point involves cases of blind, painful eyes. Surgeons need to be wary of a certain low incidence of unknown intraocular tumors that may have been the cause of the vision loss.[5,6] Careful ultrasound evaluation and a well-documented history leading up to the blind, painful eye are important steps before proceeding to an evisceration.

As a final clinical consideration, you have to consider how evisceration and enucleation affect sympathetic ophthalmia. After a ruptured globe has been repaired but deemed to have no light perception, both eviscerations and enucleations have been done as prophylaxis against sympathetic ophthalmia in the contralateral eye. Some believe that evisceration is not as protective as enucleation, but the literature does not convincingly support this hypothesis.[1,7,8] Part of the difficulty is the rarity of this complication in general, requiring decades to collect a few cases. However, careful review of published papers shows that, in fact, there are a small but comparable number of cases of sympathetic ophthalmia reported after either procedure, but you have to go back 100 years to find them.[9-13] Almost all the cases involved prolonged periods between the rupture, surgical repair, and globe removal; had clear evidence of residual uveal tissue in the orbit; or did not have specific documentation. None of these cases clearly met the current standard of care, including repair of the globe within 24 hours and evisceration/enucleation within 10 days with careful removal of uveal tissue. The sympathetic ophthalmia easily could have occurred from the prolonged uveal exposure rather than from an issue with the evisceration or enucleation.

It has also been proposed that eviscerations may actually induce sympathetic ophthalmia because of residual uveal tissue remaining after the procedure. There is little evidence to support this idea, but one case report does mention a patient with a long history of a blind eye that was eviscerated 60 years after the original injury who developed sympathetic ophthalmia 14 weeks later.[11] Of course, during evisceration, meticulous removal of all uveal tissue is required, and as an added precaution, surgeons will often denature any potential microscopic uveal tissue embedded in the sclera by thoroughly coating the inner sclera with alcohol.

For either procedure, an orbital implant is placed at the time of surgery. The older implants are nonporous and include silicone, acrylic, and polymethyl-methacrylate (PMMA), while newer porous materials include polyethylene, hydroxyapatite, and aluminum oxide. The porous materials theoretically allow fibrovascular ingrowth that was designed to promote stability and motility. For enucleations, some porous materials can allow direct suturing of the extraocular muscles to the implant. However, you can also wrap the implant in a variety of donor tissues, like sclera or pericardium, and suture to the wrapping instead. Donor tissue, of course, raises a small concern for transmission of disease. Both classes of implants are widely used and have good long-term stability. I personally prefer nonporous implants, especially silicone, because it is smooth and soft against the surrounding tissue. In my experience, the vast majority of extruded implants that I have removed have been porous.

As for the motility issue, studies failed to show significant differences in the motility achieved with porous and nonporous implants.[14-16] Perhaps most importantly, the endpoint for these patients is not the motility of the implant but of the prosthesis, which sits anterior to the implant. A 1-mm difference in the implant moving does not likely make any difference to the prosthesis, largely because the implant and the prosthesis are not physically connected. Instead, the movement of the prosthesis mechanically depends on, and is limited by, the fornices changing as the implant moves.

One last consideration is pegging, where the implant and prosthesis are mechanically coupled. Pegging can only be performed with porous implants. This process certainly augmented the movement, but extrusion rates were largely unacceptable because pegging required creating a defect in the careful multilayer closure over the orbital implant. I do not use pegging and a recent survey of ASOPRS members suggests that this is a general trend. However, even though the technique is not generally used at this time, further innovation is ongoing to make this a more tenable option. If the extrusion issues with pegging are resolved, porous implants could become considerably more popular.

Summary

Evisceration and enucleation are both good procedures from a technical point of view, and either can be done in most clinical scenarios.[17] Exceptions include evisceration with intraocular tumors and possibly enucleation with endophthalmitis. At the moment, I personally prefer evisceration due to its simplicity, efficiency, and the good cosmetic results.[3] Most importantly, based on the current literature, the concern of sympathetic ophthalmia following evisceration seems unfounded.

References

1. Levine MR, Pou CR, Lash RH. The 1998 Wendell Hughes Lecture. Evisceration: is sympathetic ophthalmia a concern in the new millennium? *Ophthal Plast Reconstr Surg.* 1999;15(1):4-8.
2. Shah RD, Singa RM, Aakalu VK, Setabutr P. Evisceration and enucleation: a national survery of practice patterns in the United States. *Ophthalmic Surg Lasers Imaging.* 2012;43(5):425-430.

3. Phan LT, Hwang TN, McCulley TJ. Evisceration in the modern age. *Middle East Afr J. Ophthalmol.* 2012;19(1):24-33.
4. Timothy NH, Freilich DR, Linberg JV. Evisceration versus enucleation from the ocularist's perspective. *Ophthal Plast Reconstr Surg.* 2003;19(6):417-420.
5. Eagle RC Jr, Grossniklaus HE, Syed N, Hogan RN, Lloyd WC 3rd, Folberg R. Inadvertent evisceration of eyes containing uvula melanoma. *Arch Ophthalmol.* 2009;127:141-145.
6. Rath S, Honavar SG, Naik MN, Gupta R, Reddy VA, Vemuganti GK. Evisceration in unsuspected intraocular tumors. *Arch Ophthalmol.* 2010;128:372-379.
7. Bilyk J. Enucleation, evisceration, and sympathetic ophthalmia. *Curr Opin Ophthalmol.* 2000;11(5):372-386.
8. du Toit N, Motala MI, Richards J, Murray AD, Maitra S. The risk of sympathetic ophthalmia following evisceration for penetrating eye injuries at Groote Schuur Hospital. *Br J Ophthalmol.* 2008;92(1):61-63.
9. Freidlin J, Pak J, Tessler HH, Putterman AM, Goldstein DA. Sympathetic ophthalmia after injury in the Iraq War. *Ophthal Plast Reconstr Surg.* 2006;22(2):133-134.
10. Green RW, Maumenee AE, Sander TE, Smith ME. Sympathetic uveitis following evisceration. *Trans Am Acad Ophthalmol Otolaryngol.* 1972;76:625-644.
11. Griepentrog GJ, Lucarelli MJ, Albert DM, Nork TM. Sympathetic ophthalmia following evisceration: a rare case. *Ophthal Plast Reconstr Surg.* 2005;21(4):316-318.
12. Dreyer WB Jr, Zegarra H, Zakov ZN, Gutman FA. Sympathetic ophthalmia. *Am J Ophthalmol.* 1981;92(6):816-823.
13. Ruedemann AD Jr. Sympathetic ophthalmia after evisceration. *Am J Ophthalmol.* 1964;57:770-790.
14. Colen TP, Paridaens DA, Lemij HG, Mourits MP, van Den Bosch WA. Comparison of artificial eye amplitudes with acrylic and hydroxyapatite spherical enucleation implants. *Ophthalmology.* 2000;107(10):1889-1894.
15. Custer PL, Trinkaus KM, Fornoff J. Comparative motility of hydroxyapatite and alloplastic enucleation implants. *Ophthalmology.* 1999;106(3):513-516.
16. González-Candial M, Umaña MA, Galvez C, Medel R, Ayala E. Comparison between motility of biointegratable and silicone orbital implants. *Am J Ophthalmol.* 2007;143(4):711-712.
17. O'Donnell BA, Kersten R, McNab A, Rose G, Rosser P. Enucleation versus evisceration. *Clin Experiment Ophthalmol.* 2005;33(1):5-9.

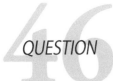
How Should I Manage Congenital Anophthalmos/Microphthalmos?

Danny Ng, FRCS, MPH and
David T. Tse, MD, FACS

What are your concerns when managing a patient with anophthalmos or micropthalmos? Is there anything to offer patients?

Congenital anophthalmos is a rare disease with an incidence of 0.2 to 0.6 per 10,000 births.[1] This condition occurs when there is complete failure of budding of the optic vesicle or early arrest of its development with subsequent degeneration. Congenital microphthalmos results from incomplete invagination of the optic vesicle into the optic cup or defective closure of the embryonic fissure of the optic vesicle.[2]

Clinical Evaluation

Initial history taking will focus on trying to make a diagnosis by establishing any other ocular or systemic features, and identifying etiological factors, in particular any relevant gestational factors or family history of other ocular or systemic abnormalities. Environmental factors have been implicated, including gestational infections, maternal vitamin A deficiency, fever, hyperthermia, exposure to x-rays, solvent misuse, and exposure to drugs like thalidomide, warfarin, and alcohol.[3,4]

The child may already be known to have other comorbidities, requiring active management by other subspecialists at this stage. While searching for any associated systemic abnormalities, particular attention is paid to the face, including ear and palate, the cardiac system, genital anomalies, feeding difficulties that might indicate esophageal abnormality, and metabolic disturbances, which may indicate pituitary underaction. A referral plan is then made depending on any systemic abnormality concerns.

The principal manifestations of congenital anophthalmia or microphthalmia are minified eyelids with abbreviated palpebral and bulbar conjunctivae and ipsilateral hypoplasia of the

Kersten RC, McCulley TJ, eds. *Curbside Consultation in Oculoplastics:*
49 Clinical Questions, Second Edition (pp 235-240).
© 2016 Taylor & Francis Group.

bony orbit. It is imperative to examine both eyes because in cases of unilateral anophthalmia or microphthalmia, the fellow eye may show other subtle abnormalities such as coloboma, optic nerve hypoplasia, retinal dystrophy, or cataract. In cases of microphthalmia, ultrasonography of the eye and orbit is performed to determine the internal structures of the eye, axial length, and the presence of an ocular remnant or cyst, which may not be immediately apparent.

Children with even severe microphthalmia may have some vision, and it is important to assess the level of visual potential of the affected eye with electrodiagnostic tests in initial evaluation to assure the parents and to guide the management approach. A flash visual evoked potential (VEP) will establish if any vision is present; a pattern VEP may yield information on acuity and optic nerve dysfunction, and an electroretinogram will identify retinal dysfunction.

In addition to orbital ultrasound and electrodiagnostic tests, I recommend neuroimaging for the child because many conditions that affect ocular development also affect brain development, particularly inspecting the midline structures, the hippocampus, and periventricular structures. Magnetic resonance imaging (MRI) is preferable to computed tomography (CT) scanning because there is higher resolution of the structures of interest and no radiation exposure. Orbital CT remains a crucial tool for determining orbital volume disparity in congenital anophthalmos, and it is important for the orbital surgeon and radiologist to work together to minimize the radiation dose to children while maintaining diagnostic image quality. Radiologists should reduce radiation exposure as low as possible by using exposure settings customized for children. Surgeons who prescribe CT imaging to assess orbital bone response to orbital tissue expander stimulation continually should assess its use on a case-by-case basis and use it prudently. Although MRI is less ideal for bone evaluation, whenever possible, MRI could be considered to monitor socket growth.

Moreover, I may order a renal ultrasound given the association between eye and renal anomalies. I will exclude intrauterine infections including congenital rubella, varicella, toxoplasma gondii, herpes simplex virus, and cytomegalovirus. In addition, early assessment of hearing is particularly important to allow prompt intervention in the case of abnormality. I will also ask other family members to come for an eye exam to look for related ocular pathology because this may provide a clue to likely diagnosis or inheritance pattern. Genetics assessment will include chromosome analysis and testing of SOX2 and OTX2 genes.[5,6] I refer the patient and family to genetic counseling for identifying a molecular cause or syndromal diagnosis, which may alter prognosis, medical management, anticipatory guidance, and reproductive risk.

Management

The ideal timing for the initial orbital tissue expander implantation in a hypoplastic juvenile orbit has yet to be determined, but it must be individualized. The rehabilitation principle teaches that simultaneous management of both soft tissue hypoplasia and asymmetric bone growth must be coordinated, and guided by the principle that application of sustained biomechanical force to the craniofacial skeleton can achieve bone growth.[7-9] Prompt expansion of minified eyelids and contracted fornices with acrylic forniceal conformers by an ocularist should begin shortly after birth and should not be delayed. Insertions of progressively enlarging forniceal conformers aim to stretch the minified eyelids and to recruit forniceal conjunctiva. In cases in which conjunctival expansion has been suboptimal or not yet initiated, placement of an expander of any kind centrally in the orbit will compromise the forniceal expansion process by limiting the space for a posterior stretching of the conjunctiva directed by the conformer. Therefore, it is necessary to allow sufficient time for soft tissue expansion and to recruit conjunctiva centrally before beginning orbital expansion. I have waited up to 2 years for soft tissue expansion to occur before beginning the orbital bony volume expansion process.

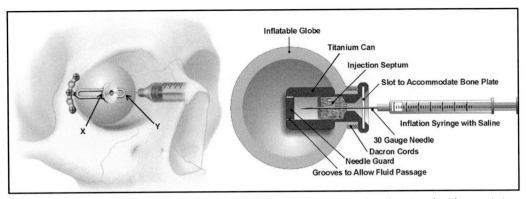

Figure 46-1. Schematic diagram of the integrated orbital tissue expander. (Reprinted with permission from Tse DT, Abdulhafez M, Orozco MA, Tse JD, Azab AO, Pinchuk L. Evaluation of an integrated orbital tissue expander in congenital anophthalmos: report of preliminary clinical experience. *Am J Ophthal.* 2011;151:470-482. © 2011 Elsevier.)

Three types of orbital expanders are available to clinicians to address the congenital orbital volume deficit problem: hard spherical implants, inflatable soft tissue expanders, and hydrogel expander implants. The hard acrylic implants require serial surgical exchanges of discrete and increasing size of spheres, thus incurring multiple anesthesias and repeated trauma to the conjunctiva.[10] Despite the arduous process of serial replacements, volume disparity remains apparent, and additional expansion may be required.[10] The inflatable soft tissue expanders are another option, but adaptation for orbital expansion is time-consuming, invasive, and technically difficult in an infant.[10,11] The principal challenges lie in controlling the direction of expansion and maintaining expander fixation within the orbit to exert sustained omnidirectional expansion pressure. Frequently, uncontrolled forward protrusion of the expander will displace the conformer or extrude early to compromise the fornix expansion process.[10-12] Hydrogel expander implants are the third option. These implantable spheres can absorb up to 2000% of their weight in water and can increase up to 30 times their original volume.[13,14] However, as the hydrogel implant reaches its equilibrium water content, the expansion forces are reduced substantially and bony stimulation ceases.[14] Further, the requisite periodic exchanges to a larger-diameter hydrogel sphere to maintain pressure holds little advantage over the conventional method of serial replacement with hard spheres of known geometry.[13]

Stimulation of orbital bone growth in congenital anophthalmos carries a significant biomedical and clinical burden. I designed an integrated orbital tissue expander to address the shortcomings of the conventional orbital expansion options and to reduce the number of surgeries (Figure 46-1).[15,16] We conducted a proof-of-concept study in an anophthalmic feline model that convincingly demonstrated that sustained application of biomechanical force to the craniofacial skeleton by serial inflation of an orbital tissue expander can lead to socket expansion. Integrated orbital tissue expander insertion is my preferred method to stimulate bony volume expansion in congenital anophthalmos.

An orbital tissue expander placement procedure is performed with the patient under general anesthesia. A transconjunctival entry into the orbit is avoided except in removing a preexisting implant so as to avoid wound dehiscence during expansion or to delay the concurrent fornix expansion. The procedure begins with a 1-cm horizontal skin incision over the lateral canthus directed toward the orbital rim (Figure 46-2A). A curvilinear periosteal incision over the lateral orbital rim is dissected to expose a broad area of the bone to accommodate the crossbar of the T-plate. The periorbita is dissected off of the lateral wall, and a 2-cm transverse incision is made at the mid orbit to provide a portal of entry for implant insertion. A Stevens scissor is introduced into the center

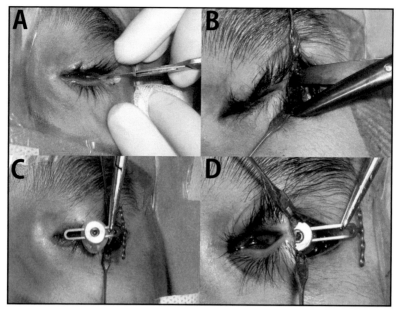

Figure 46-2. Orbital tissue expander placement in a congenital anophthalmos patient. (Reprinted with permission from Tse DT, Abdulhafez M, Orozco MA, Tse JD, Azab AO, Pinchuk L. Evaluation of an integrated orbital tissue expander in congenital anophthalmos: report of preliminary clinical experience. *Am J Ophthal.* 2011;151:470-482. © 2011 Elsevier.)

of the orbit, and the blades are widened to spread the intraconal orbital tissues to create a pocket to accommodate the expander (Figure 46-2B). An intact layer of conjunctiva is preserved to serve as a tissue barrier over the expander. A bone plate is selected and bent 90 degrees at the junction between the crossbar and the shaft using a pair of bending pliers. The orbital tissue expander is coupled to the T-plate in the slotted tunnel. Before insertion into the orbit, the expander is inflated with sterile saline to confirm its integrity. Fluid and air are aspirated from the expander to collapse the balloon to its minimal size (Figure 46-2C) to facilitate its insertion through the periorbital opening (Figure 46-2D). After the implant is positioned in the center of the orbit, the crossbar of the T-plate is maneuvered to rest over the lateral bony rim. A high-speed drill with a drill bit length of 5 mm and a diameter of 0.76 mm is used to create the drill holes. The T-plate is then secured into position with three 1-mm diameter, 5-mm long screws (Figure 46-3A).

After securing the T-plate in position, a 30-gauge needle attached to a 1- to 3-mL syringe is inserted into the injection chamber under direct view of the injection port (Figure 46-3B). Sterile normal saline is injected slowly to inflate the expander until the T-plate begins to bend outward (Figure 46-3C). In most cases, the expander is inflated with 3.0 cm^3 fluid, which is equivalent to the insertion of an 18-mm static acrylic implant. To verify that the injected fluid volume is retained, the thumb over the plunger is released, allowing the backpressure in the expander to raise the plunger and refill the syringe with the same fluid volume injected. The periosteum is closed over the cross bar of the T-plate with 5-0 polyglactin sutures. The skin incision is closed with absorbable sutures (Figure 46-3D).

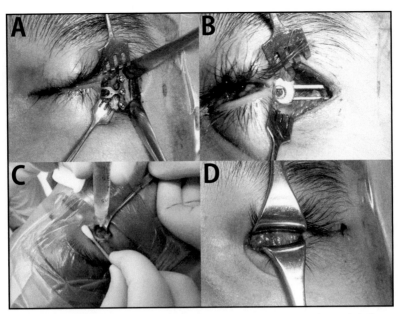

Figure 46-3. Orbital tissue expander placement in a congenital anophthalmos patient. (Reprinted with permission from Tse DT, Abdulhafez M, Orozco MA, Tse JD, Azab AO, Pinchuk L. Evaluation of an integrated orbital tissue expander in congenital anophthalmos: report of preliminary clinical experience. *Am J Ophthal.* 2011;151:470-482. © 2011 Elsevier.)

Long-Term Management

Because the expander is inserted into the orbit through a lateral canthal incision, the intact conjunctival surface permits the simultaneous wearing of a fornix conformer immediately. Second inflation is usually performed 4 to 6 months after implantation and under strict sterile protocol. Patient's prosthesis and socket are examined under anesthesia yearly to look for thinning of the overlying conjunctiva and for signs of orbital tissue expander deflation. The orbital tissue expander inflation is continued until a final volume of 4 to 5 cm^3 is reached or until the T-plate begins to bend forward to tent up the conjunctiva. The duration of implant expansion and timing for orbital tissue expander exchange to a permanent static implant should be guided by achieving the surgical objectives of orbital volume equality with the contralateral side and improvement of the hemifacial skeleton and periocular soft tissue growth.

References

1. Tucker S, Jones B, Collin JRO. Systemic anomalies in 77 patients with congenital anophthalmos or microphthalmos. *Eye.* 1996;10:310–314.
2. Fuhrmann S. Eye morphogenesis and patterning of the optic vesicle. *Curr Top Dev Biol.* 2010;93:61–84.
3. Dolk H, Busby A, Armstrong BG, Walls PH. Geographical variation in anophthalmia and microphthalmia in England, 1988–94. *BMJ.* 1998;317:905-909.
4. O'Keefe M, Webb M, Pashby RC, Wagman RD. Clinical anophthalmos. *Br J Ophthalmol.* 1987;71:635-638.

5. Matsushima D, Heavner W, Pevny LH. Combinatorial regulation of optic cup progenitor cell fate by SOX2 and PAX6. *Development*. 2011;138:443-454.
6. Schilter KF, Schneider A, Bardakjian T, et al. OTX2 microphthalmia syndrome and delineation of a phenotype. *Clin Genet*. 2011;79:158-168.
7. Heinz GW, Nunery WR, Cepela MA. The effect of maturation on the ability to stimulate orbital growth using tissue expanders in the anophthalmic cat orbit. *Ophthalmic Plast Reconstr Surg*. 1997;13(2):115-128.
8. Kiskaden WS, McDowell AJ, Keiser T. Results of early treatment of congenital anophthalmos. *Plast Reconstr Surg*. 1949;4(5):426-433.
9. Price E, Simon JW, Calhoun JH. Prosthetic treatment of severe microphthalmos in infancy. *J Pediatr Ophthalmol Strabismus*. 1986;23(1):22–24.
10. Tucker SM, Sapp N, Collin R. Orbital expansion of congenitally anophthalmic socket. *Br J Ophthalmol*. 1995;79(7):667–671.
11. Gossman MD, Mohay J, Roberts DM. Expansion of the human microphthalmic orbit. *Ophthalmology*. 1999;106(10):2005–2009.
12. Anderson RL. Commentary on Cepela MA, Nunery WR, Martin RT. Stimulation of orbital growth by the use of expandable implants in the anophthalmic cat orbit. *Ophthalmic Plast Reconstr Surg*. 1992;8(3):168-169.
13. Wiese KG, Vogel M, Guthoff R, Gundlach KKH. Treatment of congenital anophthalmos with self-inflating polymer expanders: A new method. *J Craniomaxillofac Surg*. 1999;27(2):72-76.
14. Gundlach KKH, Guthoff RF, Hingst VHM, Schittkowski MP, Bier UC. Expansion of the socket and orbit for congenital clinical anophthalmia. *Plast Reconstr Surg*. 2005;116(5):1214-1222.
15. Tse DT, inventor; University of Miami (Miami, FL), assignee. Integrated rigid fixation orbital expander. US Patent 6,582,465 B2, June 24, 2003.
16. Tse DT, Pinchuk L, Davis S, et al. Evaluation of an integrated orbital tissue expander in an anophthalmic feline model. *Am J Ophthalmol*. 2007;143(2):317–327.

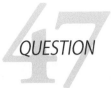
WHAT IS THE BEST APPROACH FOR TRICHIASIS?

David R. Jordan, MD, FACS, FRCSC and
Bazil Stoica, MD

What are the various methods for destroying the follicles? Can you really just laser the lashes? When would you recommend a pentagonal wedge resection? When is it best just to rotate the margin (eg, tarsotomy)? Do people still do split procedures with mucous membrane grafting?

Trichiasis refers to eyelashes that are misdirected against the eye. Common causes include eyelid inflammation (localized or diffuse; eg, blepharitis), trauma (physical or iatrogenic; eg, lid lacerations, lid biopsies, or chalazion removal), associated with cicatrizing disorders (eg, Stevens-Johnson syndrome, cicatricial pemphigoid), or localized neoplasia (eg, basal or squamous cell carcinoma). Distichiasis refers to a rare condition (generally congenital, occasionally acquired) in which an extra row of lashes arises from the miebomian gland orifices.

Numerous treatments have been suggested for trichiasis including epilation, electrolysis (hyfrecator, radiofrequency unit), cryotherapy, laser ablation, and several surgical procedures. Some degree of recurrence is not uncommon with any of these techniques. Our approach is to stay simple but be as effective as possible. The first step we take is to assess whether the misdirected lashes are localized to one area of the eyelid or are all across the lid. We assess the degree of lid margin inflammation, direction of the meibomian gland openings, and any degree of conjunctival inflammation or scarring. We also look for anterior migration of the mucocutaneous junction indicating some degree of marginal entropion. We check to see if there are any lashes arising from the meibomian gland openings (distichiaisis) or if the eyelid skin may be pushing the lashes against the cornea (epiblepharon). Keep in mind that neoplasia involving the eyelid margin may also cause trichiasis as an early sign of their presence (Figure 47-1). Subtle ulceration, telangiectasia, or lid notching are other clues to watch for but may not come until later.

If there is simply one or two inturned lashes and it is the patient's first visit with no previous history of trichiasis, we often make a note of the location of the lashes, epilate them, and inform

Kersten RC, McCulley TJ, eds. *Curbside Consultation in Oculoplastics:*
49 Clinical Questions, Second Edition (pp 241-244).
© 2016 Taylor & Francis Group.

Figure 47-1. Focal trichiasis. This patient presented with focal trichiasis involving two lashes in the mid-position of the right lower eyelid. Because there was also a slight notch in the lower eyelid, a wedge excision was performed, which identified squamous cell carcinoma in situ.

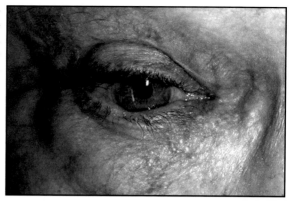

the patient of their possible recurrence and need for additional treatment. If there is any eyelid inflammation (blepharitis) associated with the area of inturned lashes, a lid hygiene routine may be suggested for nighttime that might include lid cleansing and the application of an antibiotic eye ointment (eg, erythromycin, bacitracin, fucithalmic ointment). A follow-up is scheduled for about 8 to 12 weeks to check for recurrence because manual epilation is generally a short-term solution.

If the lashes return and are less than 6 to 8 in number, our procedure of choice is argon laser ablation.[1] This is a simple procedure and highly effective (<5% recurrence). In addition to topical anesthesia (eg, tetracaine, proparacaine eye drops), local infiltration of the eyelid (2% xylocaine with epinephrine 1:100,000 mixed 50:50 with bacteriostatic saline) is used. The argon laser is turned on to the yellow/green or blue/green setting, 1300 to 1500 milliwatts, 0.3 to 0.5 seconds, 100-micron spot size. If the lashes are on the lower lid, the patient is asked to look up, the lower lid is gently rolled outward with a cotton-tipped applicator, and the laser application is applied directly down the lash root. A white plastic protective lens may be placed over the cornea for added protection. About 6 to 8 shots will take you down to a 2-mm depth. At this point, switch to a 200-μm spot size and apply an additional 3 to 4 shots to destroy residual follicular tissue. Where possible, tissue between lashes is preserved and destruction of the tarsal plate is avoided. If the lashes are colorless, the laser will not ablate them, so paint them with a gentian violet marker and reapply the laser application. Post-laser topical polysporin eye ointment is applied; healing takes place by secondary intention.

If the argon laser is unavailable, we use radiofrequency (Ellman Surgitron, Ellman International).[2] After infiltrating the lid with local anesthesia, we turn the radiofrequency unit on to the hemo-partially rectified mode, power setting of 3.5, and attach the purple-coated insulated needle (Ellman surgical catalog #D6B.007). The insulated wire tip is placed alongside the lash root, the machine is activated, and the wire tip enters the lid for about 2 mm. Application time is typically 1 to 3 seconds, and the endpoint is reached when the follicle region is cleared of tissue. Usually, there is a 0.5-mm crater or localized pit along the path of the lash follicle. Granulation tissue fills in the defect over a few days.

Alternatives to these two techniques may include localized cryotherapy.[3] The main advantage of cryotherapy is its ability to destroy large numbers of lashes quickly. The procedure is easy to learn and quick to perform. There are several cryo tips available to use. For 1 to 2 lashes, the pinpoint or 2 mm tip works well. A double freeze thaw application is carried out (25-second application → 2-minute rethaw → 25-second application). If there is a group of 6 to 8 lashes, a broad-based tip is appropriate with the same double freeze thaw technique applied. A cautionary note with cryotherapy is that it may cause local depigmentation, induce trichiasis in adjacent areas, cause lid notching, reactivate herpes zoster, or lead to further conjunctival shrinkage with symblepharon formation—an undesirable effect, especially in those with pemphigoid or Stevens-Johnson

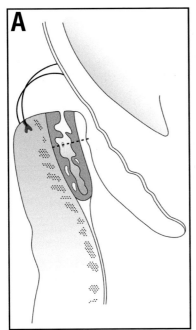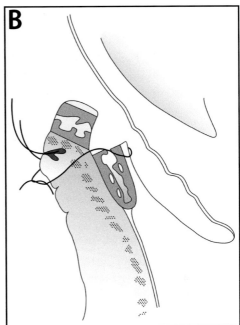

Figure 47-2. (A) The eyelid incision is made with a #15 scalpel blade about 2 to 3 mm away from the eyelid margin and only goes through the tarsal plate. (B) The double-armed 5-0 or 6-0 polyglactin sutures are passed from the conjunctival surface to the skin surface 1 to 2 mm below the lashes as shown. As they are tied, the lid margin rotates outward. Overcorrection with slight eversion is desired.

syndrome. We generally reserve cryotherapy for broad areas of the eyelid that require lash ablation (10 to 20 lashes) and prefer to use the laser or radiofrequency whenever possible.

If there is any suggestion of neoplasm (subtle ulceration of the lid margin, telangiectasia, lid notching), then a lid biopsy should be performed (pentagonal wedge excision). This not only eliminates the misdirected lashes but provides a nice biopsy specimen.

If the trichiatic lashes are located all along the lower eyelid, there is usually some degree of conjunctival cicatrization. This may be mild as in marginal entropion secondary to chronic blepharitis (posterior lid margin loses its square edge and becomes rounded, anterior migration of the mucocutaneous junction), or more obvious as in pemphigoid or Stevens-Johnson syndrome. The surgical procedure we use most often with diffuse trichiasis is a tarsotomy (Figure 47-2).[4] This procedure is done under local anesthesia. It is a simple and effective variant of tarsal fracturing (Weis procedure) with marginal rotation. It can be done all across the eyelid or just in one portion. It effectively corrects lid margin abnormalities due to mild to moderate cicatricial entropion. After incising tarsus 2 to 3 mm away from the lid margin, four to five 5-0 or 6-0 polyglactin sutures are passed from the conjunctival surface to the skin surface adjacent to the lashes (see Figure 47-2A). As the sutures are tied, the lid margin rotates outward (see Figure 47-2B).

As an alternative technique, especially if there is any degree of lid laxity, a 4-snip procedure is available.[5] A full-thickness lid resection is carried out in the area in which the trichiatic lashes are at their worst in conjunction with a tarsal fracture and lid margin rotation (Weis procedure).[5]

In more than 2 decades of oculoplastics practice within North America, the above techniques have served me well. We have not had to do any eyelid splitting at the grey line with anterior lamellar lash bulb resection, recession of the anterior lamella, or mucous membrane grafting, despite having numerous patients with conjunctival cicatricial causes to their trichiasis. The biggest problem we find with this latter technique is harvesting a thin enough piece of mucous membrane. Full-thickness buccal mucosa is quite thick. A split-thickness mucous membrane graft is much thinner and works better but there has not been a mucous membrane grafting device available for many years in North America. Recently, Storz produced one that allows harvesting of these split-thickness mucous membrane grafts from inside the lower lip, which will be beneficial when contemplating one of these more extensive procedures.

References

1. Gossman MD, Yung R, Berlin AJ, Brightwell JR. Prospective evaluation of the argon laser in the treatment of trichiasis. *Ophthal Surg.* 1992;23:183-187.
2. Kezirian GM. Treatment of localized trichiasis with radiofrequency. *Ophthal Plas Reconstr Surg.* 1993;9(4):260-266.
3. Dutton JJ, Tawfik HA, DeBacker CM, Lipham WJ. Direct internal eyelash bulb extirpation for trichiasis. *Ophthal Plast Reconstr Surg.* 2000;16(2):142-145.
4. Kersten RC, Kleiner FP, Kulwin DR. Tarsotomy for the treatment of cicatricial entropion with trichiasis. *Arch Ophthalmol.* 1992;110:714-717.
5. Allen LH. Four-snip procedure for involutional lower lid entropion: modification of Quickert and Jones procedures. *Can J Ophthalmol.* 1991;26(3):139-143.

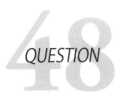
How Should I Manage My Patients With Bell's Palsy?

Andrew G. Lee, MD

What are the current thoughts on the etiology of Bell's palsy? Should patients be treated with steroid or antiviral therapy?

Bell's palsy (BP) is a term used to describe an idiopathic, isolated, acute, peripheral facial paresis. An ophthalmologist might be the initial point of medical contact for the patient because eye symptoms might predominate and an oculoplastic surgeon might be consulted because of the exposure keratopathy secondary to the facial palsy. I would strongly recommend not using the eponym Bell's palsy for every seventh nerve palsy as it can be misleading and once the diagnosis of BP is made it often becomes entrenched in the medical chart as an etiologic diagnosis when in fact it is idiopathic. This is especially problematic with electronic health records where old diagnoses can carry forward without modification or revision. Although typically the clinical diagnosis of BP is simple to make and most cases recover, up to 30% of BP patients are left with some residual dysfunction. Although some prior studies have suggested that BP might be caused by viral infections (eg, herpes simplex virus), it remains controversial. Because of the possibility that BP might be viral in origin, the use of both antivirals and steroids has been proposed as a treatment.

When considering the evidence for and against treatment of BP with steroids and/or antiviral therapy, the available evidence can be graded by class of study (eg, randomized, controlled clinical trial) and then a grade for a clinical recommendation can be made (eg, strong or weak) based on that evidence. In teaching my residents about applying this evidence base in a real-world clinical practice, I often refer to these levels of evidence as "must do" (Level A recommendation based on Class 1 studies), "should do" (ie, do or show just cause why you are not following the recommendation), "could do" (ie, a Level C practice option); "voodoo" (ie, unproven or unknown treatment effect), or "doo-doo" (ie, proven to be ineffective or possibly harmful).

Kersten RC, McCulley TJ, eds. *Curbside Consultation in Oculoplastics:*
49 Clinical Questions, Second Edition (pp 245-246).
© 2016 Taylor & Francis Group.

In 2001, the Quality Standards Subcommittee of the American Academy of Neurology (AAN) published an evidence-based practice guideline for the treatment of BP. This 2001 guideline concluded that "steroids were probably effective and antivirals (acyclovir) possibly effective in increasing the probability of complete facial functional recovery." In 2012, the AAN reviewed nine additional studies, two of which were Class I evidence.[1] For patients with new-onset BP, the new report concluded that "steroids are highly likely to be effective and should be offered to increase the probability of recovery of facial nerve function (2 Class I studies, Level A)." For patients with new-onset BP, antiviral agents in combination with steroids did not increase the probability of facial functional recovery by greater than 7%. Nevertheless, because of the possibility of a modest increase in recovery, BP patients might still be offered antivirals in addition to steroids (Level C). However, patients offered antiviral therapy should be "counseled that a benefit from antivirals has not been established, and, if there is a benefit, it is likely that it is modest at best."

Although steroids are effective and recommended in general, they may not be safe for an individual patient with BP in whom the risk to benefit ratio is unfavorable. One common example is the presence of steroid-related contraindications (eg, brittle diabetes mellitus, severe gastric ulcer disease, concomitant systemic infection risks). Therefore, clinicians and patients must make an informed decision about treatment on an individual basis. In addition, because the studies include only patients presenting early after palsy onset, it is difficult to make an evidence-based recommendation for patients with BP who present later in the course of their illness (eg, >1 or 2 weeks after onset).

Summary

BP might be due to a viral etiology but the role of antiviral therapy remains controversial and the term BP should be reserved for acute, idiopathic, and neurologically isolated seventh nerve palsy to avoid diagnostic confusion. Clinicians should consider corticosteroids in patients with BP but on an individual, risk to benefit basis. The use of antiviral treatment remains controversial because of modest if any benefit shown by current evidence.

Reference

1. Gronseth GS, Paduga R. Evidence-based guideline update: Steroids and antivirals for Bell palsy: Report of the Guideline Development Subcommittee of the American Academy of Neurology. *Neurology*. 2012;79(22):2209-2213.

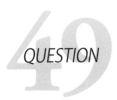

QUESTION

WHAT IS CURRENTLY RECOMMENDED FOR THE TREATMENT OF HERPES ZOSTER INVOLVING THE FACE AND EYELIDS?

Vivek R. Patel, MD

Do you recommend antiviral therapy to your patients? Do you use any topical medications? Can anything be recommended to decrease the chance of post-herpetic neuralgia?

Dermatomal involvement along the ophthalmic division of the trigeminal nerve due to herpes zoster virus (HZV) reactivation is a relatively common presentation to the ophthalmologist. The propensity for ocular surface and uveal involvement typically results in a semi-urgent consultation to an ophthalmologist. Patients typically present with a vesicular eruption along the V1 territory, with variable eyelid and ocular involvement. This chapter will summarize a treatment approach for these patients and will highlight some important considerations in their management.

General Considerations

Most patients with clinical manifestations of an HZV infection are aged older than 50 years. It is important to determine the overall immune status of the patient, particularly in younger individuals presenting with this condition. Chronic pharmacological immunosuppression with steroids, biologics, or other immunosuppressants, and HIV patients, all carry a heightened risk for affliction and more severe disease. Moreover, immunocompromised patients are more likely to develop disseminated zoster (eg, pulmonary, meningovascular, multiple dermatomes, cranial nerve involvement) and constitutional symptoms than immunocompetent patients. Pregnant patients also need to be identified and managed accordingly. A careful review of systems and knowledge of the patient's overall health status and background is essential.

Kersten RC, McCulley TJ, eds. *Curbside Consultation in Oculoplastics: 49 Clinical Questions, Second Edition* (pp 247-249).
© 2016 Taylor & Francis Group.

Ocular Surface Involvement

Nasociliary branch involvement often results in corneal manifestations such as superficial punctate keratitis, with or without raised mucoid plaques on the epithelial surface. Stromal keratitis and uveitis may also be seen. Most cases of keratitis require only topical lubrication because the condition is self-limited. Pseudodendrite formation and deeper involvement (stroma and uvea) typically is managed with careful use of topical steroids including fluorometholone (FML) 0.1% or prednisolone 1% drops, with monitoring of intraocular pressure and systemic antiviral coverage. Associated lesions on the side or tip of the nose can also be seen given common innervation of these regions by the nasociliary branch (Hutchinson's sign).

Conservative Measures

A number of conservative measures can be helpful in the active setting. Calamine lotion (zinc oxide with 0.5% iron oxide) or pads soaked in Burrow's solution (5% aluminum acetate dissolved in water) applied to the rash 4 to 6 times per day for 30 minutes at a time can help desiccate the lesions and reduce itching. For involvement of the eyelids and periocular tissues, it is reasonable to apply erythromycin or polymyxin ointment 3 times per day (TID) to the lesions using a cotton tip to prevent bacterial superinfection, in particular if the sores are open.

Systemic Therapy

I used to recommend antiviral medications (acyclovir 800 mg 5 times a day for 7 to 10 days; famcyclovir 500 mg TID for 7 days; or valacyclovir 1000 mg TID for 7 days) to patients who present within 72 hours of onset. More recently, evidence has suggested that patients presenting after 72 hours also benefit and I'll often offer antiviral medication to anyone with active lesions. The main rationale for systemic antiviral treatment is to reduce the viral load, promote earlier healing of lesions, and potentially (controversial) reduce the incidence of post-herpetic neuralgia (PHN). It is important to remember that a minority of patients can develop cranial neuropathies (presumed retrograde involvement at level of the cavernous sinus). These patients should receive a magnetic resonance image (MRI) scan of the orbits/cavernous sinus with and without gadolinium and continued on antivirals for 4 to 6 weeks. They should be observed over that time for further intracranial extension or systemic involvement.

Many practitioners recommend oral prednisone: 40 mg daily for 1 week followed by a 1- to 2-week taper. This is thought to possibly reduce associated pain and development of PHN. However, this is controversial with a lack of consensus. Given this, most will reserve its use for those patients with severe pain in the active phase. Certainly, steroids should not be given to immunocompromised patients and those with clear systemic contraindications.

Management as an inpatient for intravenous treatment and more in-depth evaluation is warranted for patients presenting with high fever, evidence, or suggestion of disseminated infection typically in the setting of an immunocompromised state, central nervous system involvement, or two or more dermatomes affected.[1] These patients should be co-managed with an internist and/or infectious disease specialist.

Post-herpetic Neuralgia

PHN remains one of the major sources of morbidity. Although it is controversial whether systemic treatment with antivirals or steroids reduces the rate of PHN, it is generally accepted that institution of early systemic treatment is important. A number of measures can be helpful in the treatment of this manifestation. Topical capsaicin cream applied 5 to 6 times daily can be effective, often following a few days of paradoxical increase in symptoms. Gabapentin (300 mg TID), Amitryptaline 25 mg every night at bedtime or Pregabalin 75 mg twice a day is effective in many cases. Patients who have persistent pain despite these initial steps in management may benefit from the expertise of a pain management specialist for more advanced approaches.

Prevention

Live attenuated varicella vaccine is now ubiquitously available and has led to a remarkable reduction in the rate of primary varicella infection. The Centers for Disease Control and Prevention has recommended that the vaccination should be given to all immune-competent and non-pregnant individuals aged older than 60 years, even if they have had a previous episode of zoster infection given that repeated clinical involvement can occur. The vaccine is contraindicated in patients actively undergoing immunosuppressive therapy, including chemotherapy or radiation, as well as pregnant women.

Varicella-zoster immune globulin (VZIG) is an important prevention and treatment option for patients who are at particular risk for dissemination.[2] Pregnant women, immunocompromised individuals, and neonates with evidence of active involvement should be treated with VZIG, given as soon as possible after suspected exposure.

References

1. Balfour HH Jr, Bean B, Laski OC, Ambinder RF, Myers JD, Wade JC, et al. Acyclovir halts the progression of herpes zoster in immunocompromised patients. *N Engl J Med.* 1983;308(24):1448-1453
2. Oxman MN, Levin MJ, Johnson GR, Schmader KE, Strauss SE, Gelb LD, et al. A Vaccine to prevent herpes zoster and post-herpetic neuralgia in older adults. *N Engl J Med.* 2005;352(22):2271-2284.

FINANCIAL DISCLOSURES

Dr. Gary L. Aguilar has no financial or proprietary interest in the materials presented herein.

Dr. Bishr Al Dabagh has no financial or proprietary interest in the materials presented herein.

Dr. Elizabeth A. Atchison has no financial or proprietary interest in the materials presented herein.

Dr. Michèle Beaconsfield has no financial or proprietary interest in the materials presented herein.

Dr. Linda C. Chang has no financial or proprietary interest in the materials presented herein.

Dr. William Chen has no financial or proprietary interest in the materials presented herein.

Dr. Richard Collin has no financial or proprietary interest in the materials presented herein.

Dr. Murray Cotter has no financial or proprietary interest in the materials presented herein.

Dr. Roger A. Dailey has no financial or proprietary interest in the materials presented herein.

Dr. Steven C. Dresner has no financial or proprietary interest in the materials presented herein.

Dr. Vikram D. Durairaj has no financial interest in any of the techniques or materials presented herein.

Dr. Bita Esmaeli has no financial or proprietary interest in the materials presented herein.

Dr. Daniel G. Ezra has no financial or proprietary interest in the materials presented herein.

Dr. James A. Garrity has no financial or proprietary interest in the materials presented herein.

Dr. Robert Alan Goldberg has no financial or proprietary interest in the materials presented herein.

Dr. Karl C. Golnik has no financial or proprietary interest in the materials presented herein.

Dr. Heidi M. Hermes has no financial or proprietary interest in the materials presented herein.

Dr. Marc J. Hirschbein has no financial or proprietary interest in the materials presented herein.

Dr. Catherine J. Hwang has no financial or proprietary interest in the materials presented herein.

Dr. Thomas N. Hwang has no financial or proprietary interest in the materials presented herein.

Dr. Thomas E. Johnson has no financial or proprietary interest in the materials presented herein.

Dr. David R. Jordan has no financial or proprietary interest in the materials presented herein.

Dr. James A. Katowitz has no financial or proprietary interest in the materials presented herein.

Dr. William R. Katowitz has no financial or proprietary interest in the materials presented herein.

Dr. Michael Kazim has no financial or proprietary interest in the materials presented herein.

Dr. Robert C. Kersten has no financial interest in any of the techniques or materials presented herein.

Dr. Don O. Kikkawa has no financial or proprietary interest in the materials presented herein.

Dr. Jane S. Kim has no financial or proprietary interest in the materials presented herein.

Dr. Jonathan W. Kim has no financial or proprietary interest in the materials presented herein.

Dr. Audrey C. Ko has no financial or proprietary interest in the materials presented herein.

Dr. Marcus J. Ko has no financial or proprietary interest in the materials presented herein.

Dr. Bobby S. Korn has no financial or proprietary interest in the materials presented herein.

Dr. Andrea Lora Kossler has no financial or proprietary interest in the materials presented herein.

Dr. Andrew G. Lee has no financial interest in any of the techniques or materials presented herein.

Dr. Bradford Lee has no financial or proprietary interest in the materials presented herein.

Dr. N. Grace Lee has no financial or proprietary interest in the materials presented herein.

Dr. Wendy W. Lee has received a research grant from Sciton and has consulted for Cutera and Lumenis.

Dr. Peter S. Levin has no financial or proprietary interest in the materials presented herein.

Dr. Sophie Liao has no financial or proprietary interest in the materials presented herein.

Dr. Mark J. Lucarelli has no financial or proprietary interest in the materials presented herein.

Dr. Nicholas R. Mahoney has no financial or proprietary interest in the materials presented herein.

Dr. Louise A. Mawn has no financial interest in any of the techniques or materials presented herein.

Dr. John D. McCann has no financial or proprietary interest in the materials presented herein.

Dr. Lynda V. McCulley has no financial or proprietary interest in the materials presented herein.

Dr. Timothy J. McCulley has no financial or proprietary interest in the materials presented herein.

Dr. Payam V. Morgan has no financial interest in any of the techniques or materials presented herein.

Dr. Maryam Nazemzadeh has no financial or proprietary interest in the materials presented herein.

Dr. Isaac M. Neuhaus has no financial or proprietary interest in the materials presented herein.

Dr. Danny Ng has no financial or proprietary interest in the materials presented herein.

Dr. John Nguyen has no financial interest in any of the techniques or materials presented herein.

Dr. Payal Patel has no financial or proprietary interest in the materials presented herein.

Dr. Vivek R. Patel has no financial interest in any of the techniques or materials presented herein.

Dr. W. Jordan Piluek has no financial or proprietary interest in the materials presented herein.

Dr. Jerry K. Popham has no financial or proprietary interest in the materials presented herein.

Dr. Roxana Rivera has no financial or proprietary interest in the materials presented herein.

Dr. Geoffrey E. Rose has no financial interest in any of the techniques or materials presented herein.

Dr. Stuart R. Seiff has no financial or proprietary interest in the materials presented herein.

Dr. Rona Z. Silkiss has no financial or proprietary interest in the materials presented herein.

Dr. Jennifer A. Sivak-Callcott has no financial interest in any of the techniques or materials presented herein.

Dr. Jonathan Song has no financial or proprietary interest in the materials presented herein.

Dr. Bazil Stoica has no financial or proprietary interest in the materials presented herein.

Dr. Prem Subramanian has no financial interest in any of the techniques or materials presented herein.

Dr. Timothy J. Sullivan has no financial or proprietary interest in the materials presented herein.

Dr. Chris Thiagarajah has no financial or proprietary interest in the materials presented herein.

Dr. Daniel J. Townsend has no financial or proprietary interest in the materials presented herein.

Dr. David T. Tse is the inventor of the integrated orbital tissue expander, which is assigned to the University of Miami and licensed exclusively to Innovia LLC. Dr. Tse receives royalties from the sale of the device by Innovia.

Dr. Roger E. Turbin has no financial interest in any of the techniques or materials presented herein.

Dr. Ana Carolina Victoria has no financial or proprietary interest in the materials presented herein.

Dr. Timothy S. Wang has no financial interest in any of the techniques or materials presented herein.

Dr. Michael T. Yen has no financial interest in any of the techniques or materials presented herein.

Dr. Michael K. Yoon has no financial or proprietary interest in the materials presented herein.

Dr. Siegrid S. Yu has no financial or proprietary interest in the materials presented herein.

INDEX

Printed in the United States
by Baker & Taylor Publisher Services